A CHRISTIAN MARRIAGE BOOK
52-WEEK DEVOTIONAL FOR WIVES

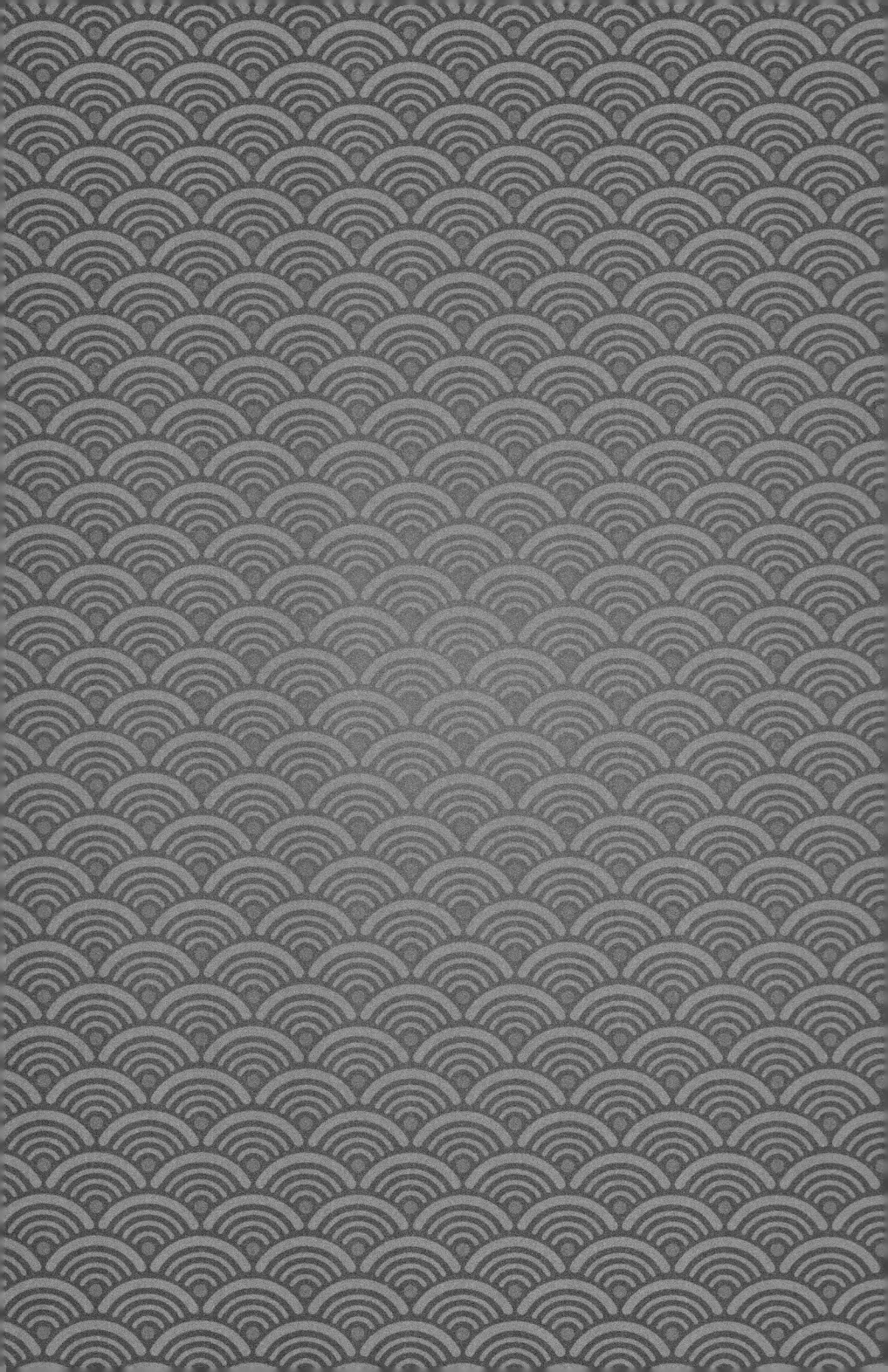

A CHRISTIAN MARRIAGE BOOK

52-WEEK
DEVOTIONAL
— *for* —
WIVES

PRAYERS AND REFLECTIONS
FOR A GOD-CENTERED MARRIAGE

TAMARA CHAMBERLAIN

ROCKRIDGE
PRESS

For general information on our other products and services or to obtain technical support, please contact our Customer Care Department within the United States at (866) 744-2665, or outside the United States at (510) 253-0500.

Rockridge Press publishes its books in a variety of electronic and print formats. Some content that appears in print may not be available in electronic books, and vice versa.

TRADEMARKS: Rockridge Press and the Rockridge Press logo are trademarks or registered trademarks of Callisto Media Inc. and/or its affiliates, in the United States and other countries, and may not be used without written permission. All other trademarks are the property of their respective owners. Rockridge Press is not associated with any product or vendor mentioned in this book.

Series Designer: Richard Tapp
Interior and Cover Designer: Angela Navarra
Art Producer: Janice Ackerman
Editor: Adrian Potts
Production Editor: Ruth Sakata Corley
Production Manager: Jose Olivera

Author photo courtesy of Hilary S. Barreto

All Scripture quotations, unless otherwise indicated, are taken from the Holy Bible, New International Version®, NIV®. Copyright ©1973, 1978, 1984, 2011 by Biblica, Inc.™ Used by permission of Zondervan. All rights reserved worldwide. www.zondervan.com. The "NIV" and "New International Version" are trademarks registered in the United States Patent and Trademark Office by Biblica, Inc.™

Paperback ISBN: 978-1-63807-207-2
eBook ISBN: 978-1-63807-589-9
R0

To my son, Titus. I love you dearly and will forever cherish the hours you spent bouncing on my lap as I wrote this book.

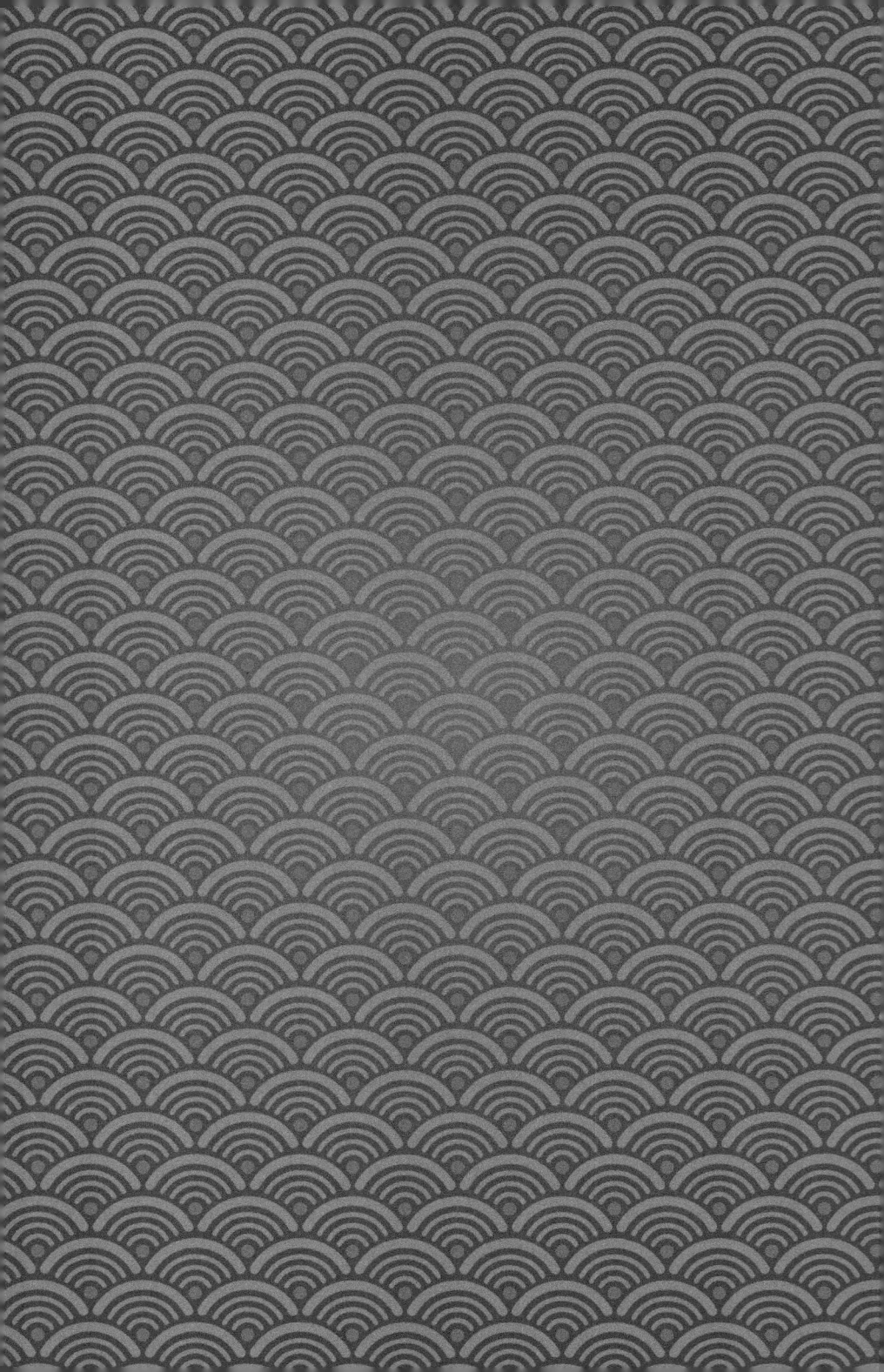

Contents

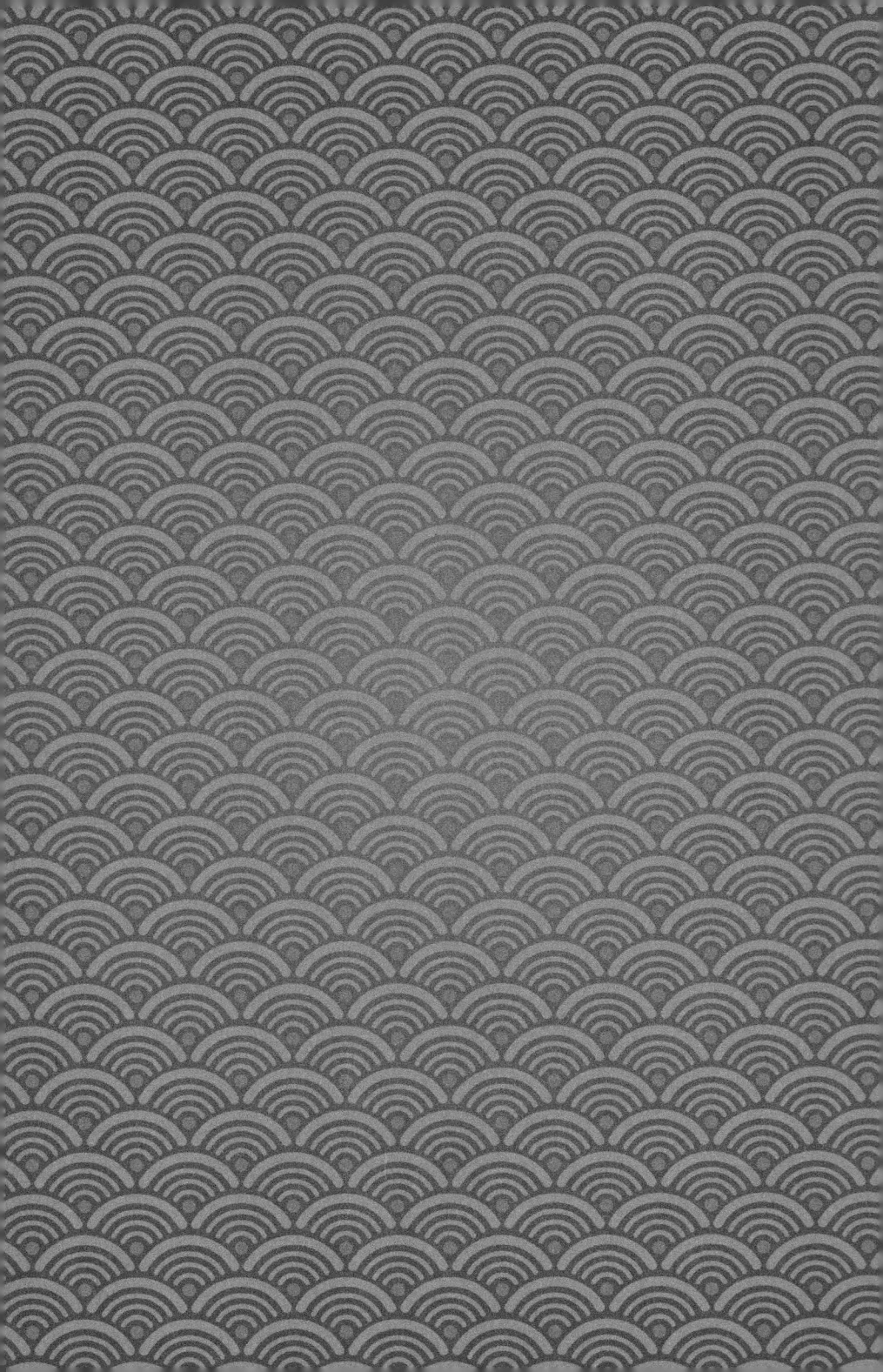

Introduction

I don't know what made you pick up this book, but I am so happy you did. Maybe this book was an engagement or wedding gift. You might be married and longing for a way to reconnect with your spouse, or maybe you'd like to see how you can grow together in your walk with God. Whatever has led you here, my prayer for you is for God to use the words on each page to show you more of his love, grace, and desire to see your marriage thrive. Whether you have been married for fifty years or two years, or are recently engaged, this book was written for you.

The heart behind this devotional is to strengthen, encourage, and equip you as you pore over the truths of Scripture that will help guide and support your marriage in ways that are useful and relevant. I will be the first to admit that I don't have it all figured out when it comes to the topic of marriage. Just like you, my husband, Dale, and I are constantly discovering, with each passing day, what it means to love each other in the way God has called us. There are seasons when loving each other comes naturally, then there are times when Dale and I are reminded of how desperately we need the strength of Jesus to love each other as he does, and I will discuss some instances of our journey in this devotional. During my four years of serving in ministry, counseling engaged couples, and standing alongside married couples, I know my experience is not uncommon.

Though the Bible was not written as a guide to maintain a long-lasting marriage, it does have a lot to say about how we can better orient our hearts and lives so we can see our marriages thrive as God intended. It is my hope not only to share my own stories and experiences about marriage with you but also to use my years of deeply studying Scripture to help encourage and strengthen your marriage. Thank you for trusting me to join you in this process.

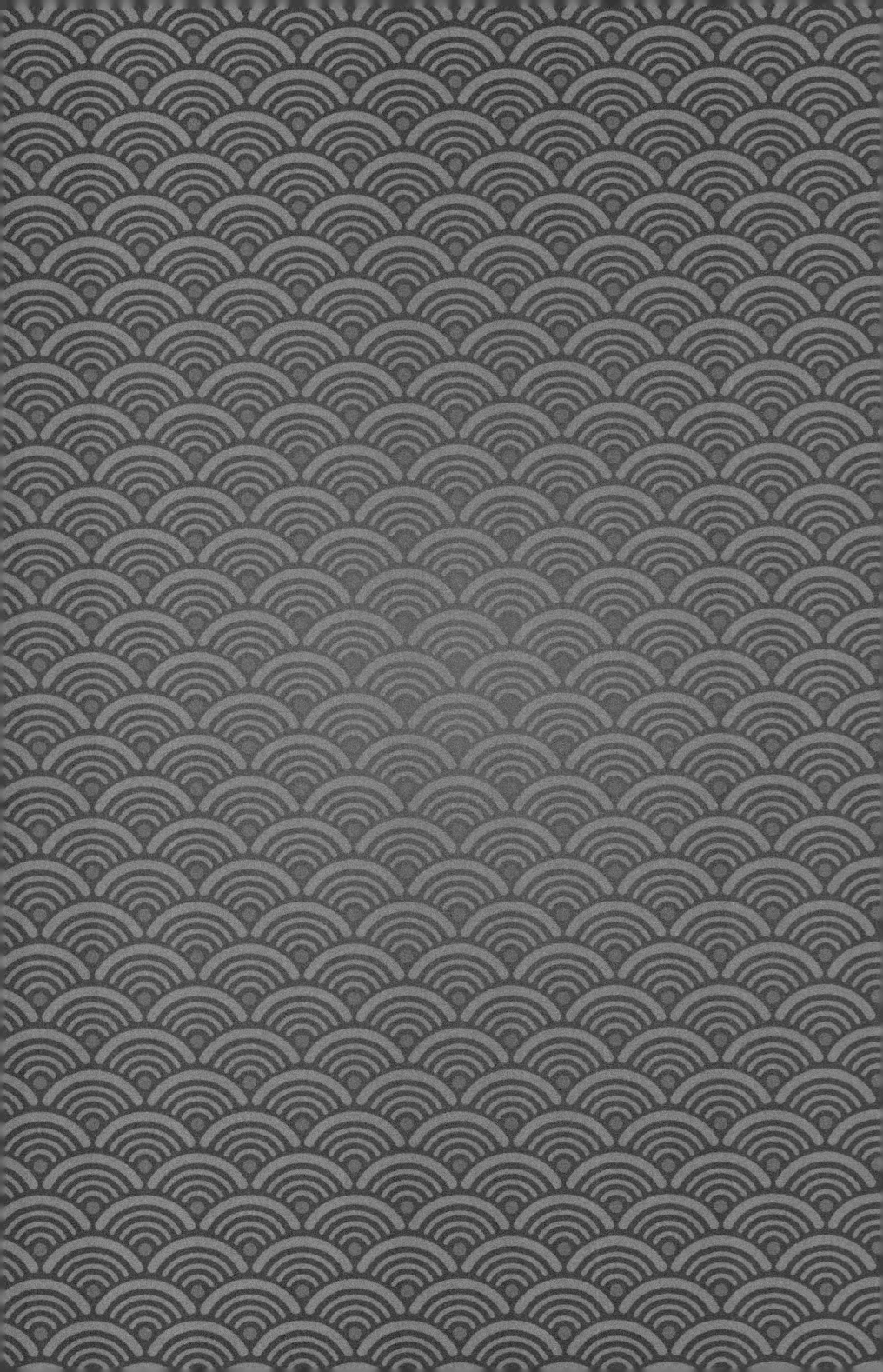

How to Use This Book

The intent of this devotional's approach is for you to use it on a weekly basis, progressing through the book from weeks 1 through 52. However, I want you to do what works best for you. I encourage you to move through the devotions based on topics that seem most relevant in your life, or even to revisit those you find most impactful. *A Christian Marriage Book—52-Week Devotional for Wives* is full of varying topics and situations that you will come across in your marriage, and it is designed to look at them from a biblical standpoint. There are many ways you can read this book—and, again, do what works best for you—but here are a few recommendations:

◆ Find a quiet space where you won't be interrupted or distracted.

◆ Have a journal or the Notes app on your phone available to write down your thoughts as you read through each devotion.

◆ Commit to taking the time to study the Scripture in each devotion and have your Bible available to read the high-lighted verses.

◆ Take an extra few minutes to engage with the final section in the devotion. This may mean adapting the prayer to fit what's in your heart, truly being honest with the reflection questions, or committing to take the suggested next steps.

◆ Bookmark the prayers to go back to again, and pray during particular situations when you need them the most.

◆ Allow the Holy Spirit to work in your heart and mind as you remember the themes and verses highlighted in each devotion.

As helpful as I pray these devotionals will be in your life, they are not intended to replace therapy or couples counseling. If you sense you have a need for professional guidance in your marriage, I encourage you to make it a top priority. It takes investment and intentionality from both spouses to build a marriage that will last, but one of the most important steps is for you to commit to doing what you can. The Lord will honor your commitment and draw you closer to himself in the process.

SHARING YOUR JOURNEY

A healthy and prosperous marriage depends on the intentionality and effort of both you and your spouse. I encourage you to find ways to bring your spouse into this process. The companion to this book, *A Christian Marriage Book—52-Week Devotional for Husbands*, can also be used to share your journey.

Regardless of the approach you take, my hope is for the devotions ahead to be used not only for your own personal growth and what you contribute to your marriage but also for sparking conversation, reflection, and prayer with each other. I hope you can find ways to step into this path together as you rely on God to love each other.

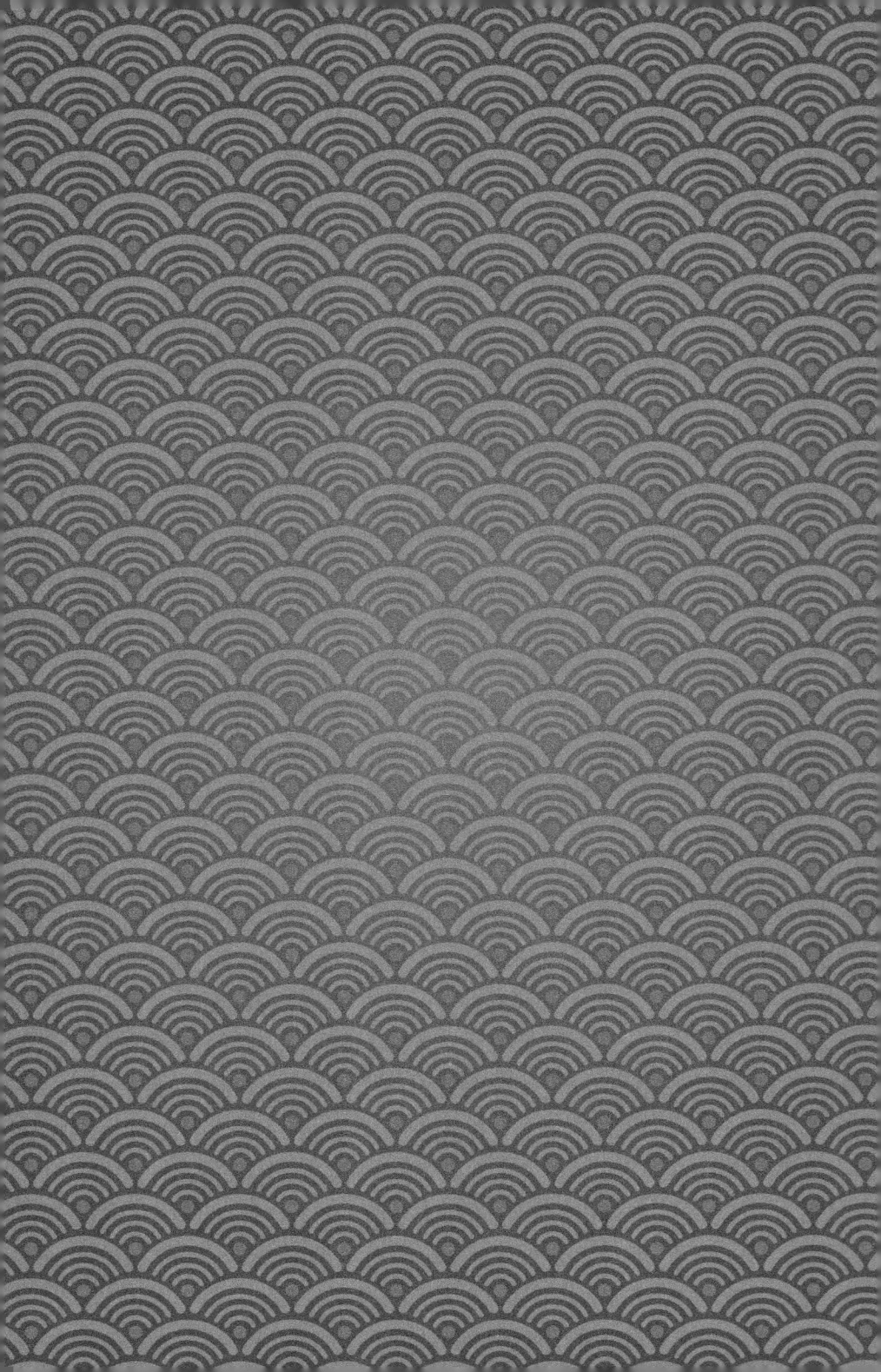

DEVOTIONALS

THE POWER OF YOUR THOUGHTS

Do not conform to the pattern of this world, but be transformed by the renewing of your mind. Then you will be able to test and approve what God's will is—his good, pleasing and perfect will.

—Romans 12:2

Out of creation, God called one man to be set apart. He was meant to live differently from the rest of the world. He was to be the beginning of God's redemption story to the world. This man, Abram, would later be called Abraham. He would leave everything he knew, travel to a new land, and faithfully follow God. The entire trajectory of Abraham's life changed forever. The way he lived, where he lived, the decisions he made, and even his relationships. Every part of who he was became centered on his relationship with God.

This is the way we are also called to live.

In order to discover what it means to carry out the various roles in your life well, you must first discover what it means to center every decision, desire, and dream on the will of God. That's why it's so important for us to take the words of Paul from Romans 12 to heart. In his letter to the Roman church, he instructs Christians on how they should live with Jesus at the center. He urges believers not to allow the world to teach them how to think and act. Instead, we are to be transformed in not only our spirit but also our mind. The Holy Spirit wants to completely transform who you are and the way you live. Often-times, transformation begins with the way we think and the perspectives we hold.

As you seek to center your marriage on God, one of the best places to begin is by praying for the Holy Spirit to use the Word of God to renew your mind. As Paul says, from here you are more able to discern and test the will of God in your life and in your marriage. Allowing your thoughts to be influenced and changed by the Holy Spirit will equip you to make decisions, sacrifices, and acts of love for the betterment of your marriage. What you allow to take root in your mind will guide the way you live. A whole life centered on God is one that is guided and directed by his will rather than the wisdom and will of the world. This week, I encourage you to actively choose to surrender your thoughts to the Holy Spirit.

Let's reflect: *Is your entire life—and are your thoughts—centered on Jesus? What or who are the top three sources of influence in how you view your marriage? Take time this week to reflect on whether or not these sources of influence are drawing your marriage closer to Jesus or further away.*

A COMMITMENT TO PRAYER

And if we know that he hears us—whatever we ask—we know that we have what we asked of him.

—1 John 5:15

I was mere months into my marriage when I found myself longing for things to be different. My husband's job had pulled him away multiple nights of the week and even on the weekends. I knew these commitments existed prior to our marriage, but having lived separately, I didn't understand the fullness of what this meant for my marriage.

As a just-married couple, I longed to have my husband home with me after work. I wanted to enjoy dinner together and unwind from our long days apart. I drove home from work one day in tears, knowing I would be going home to an empty house . . . again. I didn't know what to do because this was his livelihood. It seemed rather extreme to ask him to quit his longtime job because I didn't want to eat dinner alone.

Sometimes, there are aspects of marriage that aren't exactly what you had envisioned. They aren't necessarily full-blown dilemmas or matters to engage in conflict over. Nevertheless, marriage can bring less-than-ideal situations, and even those seemingly small areas of unmet expectations can begin to chip away at the bond you share.

It's hard to know what to do and even if a resolution can be reached. You may not be able to change the circumstance or simply move something from an unmet expectation to one that's fulfilled overnight. But what you can do is pray. I began to pray every day on my way home from work. After months of prayer, I finally began to see my heart toward the situation change. I became more understanding of my husband's obligations, and he made efforts to limit his number of weeknight commitments. God drew us closer together through the process of bringing this concern before his throne.

We should have a sense of confidence coming before God and praying for all aspects of our marriage—from the seemingly small to the overwhelmingly large. The first book of John ends with this very truth. Essentially, John is telling us that if we can be confident enough that the work of Jesus provides eternal life, then we can confidently approach God with our requests. It's important to note that John isn't depicting God as a magic genie who will make all of your dreams come true; what he's saying is that when our prayer request is in the will of God, then we know it will come to pass.

It doesn't matter how silly or trite you think your prayer requests are. God hears them. He will answer them according to his will, but approaching him confidently on behalf of your marriage will cause transformation to happen in your relationship.

Let's put it into practice: What two areas of your marriage have been on your mind? What unmet expectations, unresolved conflict, uncontrollable situations, or lack of connection have you determined? Commit to praying for these two areas for the next seven days. Begin your prayer by openly sharing your thoughts with God and asking for him to work in your marriage to change the situation.

CHOOSING GOOD FOR YOUR MARRIAGE

For we are taking pains to do what is right, not only in the eyes of the Lord but also in the eyes of man.

—2 Corinthians 8:21

I've found the discipline of dating your spouse becomes increasingly difficult with young children. There is a lot of prep work and scheduling that goes into arranging time away as a couple. For us, a weekly date night was not as practical as all of the marriage books made it seem to be. Seeing the value of intentional time together, Dale and I became creative. Every Friday after the children are in bed for the night, we order takeout from a restaurant we would normally visit for a date night, sit in our backyard, and spend a few uninterrupted hours together. I genuinely look forward to our Friday nights together.

Just as we decided to truly make this a priority in our marriage, it seemed like out of nowhere we were being invited to events on Fridays. There was a great temptation to push our date night off for the second, third, or fourth week in a row. As we began to develop the discipline of dating each other, it was important to make the decision that was right by our marriage and put our intentional time together above all else.

There are decisions you will have to make with the motivation of doing what is right for your relationship. Sometimes, choosing your marriage might feel like you are letting people down or are missing out on good opportunities. Choosing what is best for your marriage is an investment in your future and in your life.

In Paul's second letter to the church of Corinth, he explains how he is taking great pains to choose what is right before the Lord and before the people involved. This particular situation is regarding the way Paul is choosing to use the financial gifts made to his ministry by the recipients of the letter and many other Christians. He takes into consideration the full weight of how he stewards the gifts of others. He understands that it's about more than the money; it's about honoring both the Lord and those who've given. He wants to care for the relationships and the hearts of the people.

Though the topic of marriage is not what Paul's words center on, we can still find great benefit in applying them to our marriage. There is great wisdom in doing what is right by the Lord and your marriage. The daily task of making decisions on the basis of what is best for your relationship will have a compounding effect and strengthen your union. When you and your spouse think of each other during the various decisions that will affect your marriage, it will go a long way in forming a bond that can't be broken.

Let's put it into practice: Take some time this week to reflect with your spouse on a decision you've made with or without each other that has impacted your relationship. It could have been a scheduling decision or even a financial purchase. I encourage you to write down a list of two or three ways you can both be intentional about putting your marriage first.

DISCIPLINE OF GRATITUDE

Jesus asked, "Were not all ten cleansed? Where are the other nine? Has no one returned to give praise to God except this foreigner?" Then he said to him, "Rise and go; your faith has made you well."

—Luke 17:17–19

The ultimate call of every Christian is to love God and love others. Jesus was the greatest example of the lengths to which we should go to show our love for others. He came to serve those he loved.

This is the call we have in every aspect of life, but the opportunities to live this out in your marriage are endless. Because of the nature of two lives merging together into one, it becomes easy to feel taken for granted. One partner might feel like they are the one doing all of the serving, whereas the other one is doing all of the receiving.

As important as service is in your marriage, so is gratitude. Acknowledging and verbalizing your appreciation for each other goes a long way.

Jesus has never been in need of our gratitude, but he has something to say about the importance of gratitude. In the account of Luke, we read about Jesus traveling to Jerusalem. On his journey he runs into ten lepers who ask for him to heal them. He does, which is not an unexpected response. Then one turns back to literally give a shout of praise for his healing.

The story takes an interesting turn when Jesus asks after the other nine lepers. Only one came back to give praise and thanks to Jesus for his healing. One out of ten! And, to top it off, he is not familiar with Jesus's ministry. It's like the other nine assume they will be healed. Yet the one who doesn't feel entitled, doesn't feel he will automatically be healed, is most grateful.

In the daily ups and downs of a marriage, there are many times when you may both feel entitled to certain things from each other. When one of you doesn't provide these things, the other is quick to become upset. And when one of you does provide these things, the other is not equally as quick to show gratitude. Certainly, marriage is about partnering together and sharing the responsibilities of life, but you must be cautious not to grow entitled in the way you share the load. Showing your appreciation for the way you share the daily tasks of life is important.

It is far better to be like the one leper who runs back to praise Jesus for his healing than the nine who just assume they'll receive Jesus's healing power.

Developing a heart of gratitude rather than entitlement will strengthen your marriage. Verbally expressing gratitude in the moment will draw you closer together. You might even be surprised how this intentional action changes the dynamic of your marriage.

Let's put it into practice: Over the next few days, be intentional about noticing the way you help each other. Regardless of how big, small, expected, or unexpected the task is, offer thanks. Verbally say, "Thank you," or "I appreciate you," to each other.

KINDNESS WITH NO STRINGS ATTACHED

Let us not become weary in doing good, for at the proper time we will reap a harvest if we do not give up. Therefore, as we have opportunity, let us do good to all people, especially to those who belong to the family of believers.

—Galatians 6:9–10

As a kid, I found great joy in slipping notes of encouragement into my mom's purse or putting my clip art skills to work and decorating a two-page letter filled with reasons why I appreciated her. This expression of love took on different forms once I was married. I enjoyed picking up something extra when I was running errands to let Dale know I was thinking of him or leaving him notes in his car reminding him that I loved him.

I don't know at what point I stopped doing these things for him, but as I sit here and write this, I can't think of the last time I did either one of those things for him. In the beginning days of my marriage, I was so excited to find small and meaningful ways to show Dale that I loved and appreciated him. As life got busier and our two children began to require so much more of me, I slowly let these small and intentional acts of kindness slip away.

In Paul's letter to the church in Galatia, he's reminding them to never grow weary in doing good. He wants them to do good for others when it's no longer trendy and no one's watching. If he were to speak these words today, he would tell us to go out of our way to be kind to others even when it's not being recorded to share on social media. We should seize every opportunity to do good for others and to care for others. This is truer in a marriage.

There will be moments in your marriage when you or your spouse will have the opportunity to show kindness or thoughtfulness without it being reciprocated in that moment. Both partners should be mindful of ways big and small to show love to each other. It might look like your spouse giving you a few hours alone after a stressful week; or maybe you can be the one to make the coffee if you know they have a late start to the day.

Let the words of Paul be the anthem to your marriage to never grow weary in doing good for your relationship. The Lord will honor your faithfulness and continue to make you more like him through your willingness.

Let's put it into practice: Each day this week, challenge yourselves to find one act of kindness or a thoughtful gesture to do for each other. Truly find ways to do good with no strings attached, and remember Paul's words as your marriage's anthem.

BEING COMMITTED TO YOUR WORDS

Whatever your lips utter you must be sure to do, because you made your vow freely to the Lord your God with your own mouth.

—Deuteronomy 23:23

There is great security within the covenant of marriage. It is designed to be a commitment you honor and treasure until your last days. With this sense of security can come the temptation to be neglectful.

I've had to catch myself from becoming too lax in my relationship. The two of us might agree that we need a weekend free of commitments, then I add an event to our calendar because I know my husband will *understand*. Of course he will understand, but that doesn't mean I shouldn't take our agreement seriously. It might seem relatively harmless to change certain things we agreed upon. This becomes harmful to your relationship when it becomes the norm rather than the exception.

The Book of Deuteronomy is filled with the laws God called on the Israelite people to live by. He wanted them to live differently than the people around them, and in order to do that, he needed to instruct them on what exactly that looked like.

As Christians who are saved by Jesus, we are not bound to the laws in the way the Israelites were. But there are many aspects of the law that we should still heed in our lives today. The last few verses of Deuteronomy 23 are those such verses. They lay out the importance of being true to your word. This principle can be seen in many places throughout Scripture, but in

Deuteronomy we actually read it as a command to God's people. He takes being a person of your word seriously, and so should we.

Regardless of how understanding you and your spouse are of each other, neither of you should use this as a reason not to be true to your word. As the verse says, "Whatever your lips utter you must be sure to do."

Maintaining a high regard for follow-through in a marriage allows you to trust and depend on each other. It also shows a great sense of respect. If either of you constantly retracts or disregards the promises you've made, then the other will have a hard time knowing that they are valued. Placing a high regard on keeping your word is one of the most valuable ways of expressing love for each other.

Let's reflect: When was the last time you made a verbal commitment or agreement within your marriage, or elsewhere, and didn't keep it? Did you think it wasn't a big deal not to follow through with what you said? How can you become more intentional about being true to what you say?

SEEING THE GOOD IN EACH OTHER

*Be devoted to one another in love. Honor one
another above yourselves.*

—Romans 12:10

We've all met the mom whose default response to a negative report of her child is, "My little Johnny would never . . ." She just couldn't possibly believe her sweet angel would be anything other than kind. As a mother, she unequivocally sees the good in her child at all times.

Seeing nothing but the good in others is what Paul means when he calls Christians to be devoted to one another in love. The way we do that is by showing honor to others. In the original Greek, the last half of this verse could be literally translated as taking the lead of one another in honor. Paul is calling us to outdo one another in honor, and by doing this we remain devoted to one another in love.

A love like this is the kind we need to have in a marriage. Not a foolish kind of love, but a prudent love that continues to see the good. You and your spouse should find opportunities to lead the way by showing honor for each other. This looks like constantly keeping the good qualities of the other at the forefront of your mind. You might not always find ways to honor each other in action and deed, but there is always an opportunity to honor each other in the judgment of the mind.

When you live with someone, their flaws great and small are on full display. As the years of marriage pass, it may even start to seem that the flaws eclipse the good qualities. Your point of view becomes focused on the characteristics and tendencies you wish were different. This is a very natural habit for humans and spouses. Yet the kind of love Jesus calls us to have for each other is a devoted and genuine love, even when you see a person in their truest form. This is a discipline you will need to practice over and over again. When a certain behavior or situation frustrates you, pause to see the good in each other. This practice will go a long way in developing a discipline of loving each other radically.

Allow the best-case scenario to be the default when it comes to how you view each other in your marriage. This is what it looks like to truly honor and love as described in this week's verse. Think the best of your spouse when they forget to pick up dinner on the way home, take four months to change the batteries in the smoke detector, snap when you ask a simple question, or continue to check out after getting home from work.

I am not suggesting you ignore issues within your marriage and push them aside for the sake of honoring each other. It's healthy to choose to talk about the difficulties or disconnect in your marriage while still loving and honoring your life partner. This may not always bring about resolution, so I encourage you to seek advice from a counselor or pastor in such cases.

Let's pray: Father, give me eyes to see the good in my spouse. Show me ways to honor them in the midst of any shortcomings. Help us honor and love each other with radical love. Amen.

YOUR GREATEST SUPERPOWER

The words of the reckless pierce like swords, but the tongue of the wise brings healing.

—Proverbs 12:18

In your possession is the single greatest weapon to build up or tear down your marriage—your words.

King Solomon, the writer of Proverbs, understood how powerful words are. When used in a thoughtful and caring way, our words can be a healing balm to a person's greatest pain. When used recklessly and carelessly, they can inflict deep pain and sorrow. It would serve well your marriage, and your life in general, to heed the advice of King Solomon.

The way you talk to and about your spouse has the power to strengthen or destroy your marriage. With each negative and sarcastic remark, you are slowly chipping away at the foundation of what holds you two together. But every loving, affirming, and caring word equally has the power to fortify and knit the two of you closer together.

Since the very beginning of my relationship with my husband, we vowed to be cautious about how we spoke to each other. My husband had a verbally abusive childhood, and I hoped our relationship would be the opposite of that in every way. I want to encourage Dale and treat him with dignity, value, and worth in the way that I speak to him and about him. I don't always get this right, but this has become a high value in our marriage. Slowly, we've created a culture that simply won't allow us to speak to each other in a demeaning, hostile, or degrading way.

I have experienced relationships where the principle of honesty became a pass to ruthlessly hurl hurtful words. I think this is a common misunderstanding of what it means to be a person of honesty and integrity. We should never give ourselves the freedom to painfully pierce the hearts and minds of our loved ones with our words. Love should not be sacrificed on the altar of "honesty." We must find ways to be honest without compromising love.

Your marriage will no longer be a safe or secure place if you lack regard for the way you speak with each other. It's important to cultivate a culture of love and safety within your relationship, and that starts with the way you allow yourselves to speak with and about each other.

We should never desire to inflict pain or hurt, regardless of the ways we've been hurt. As a couple, you see the good, bad, and ugly in each other. You know the exact words that will cut each other the deepest. You also know the words to say that will bring encouragement and security to each other. God has called you to love each other in both the good and the bad, which means choosing to speak life and healing over each other rather than harm and pain.

Let's reflect: *How often do you speak words of encouragement and care to your loved ones? How often do you remind them of the ways they are lacking or fall short? Use this week to take stock of how often your words bring life and how often they bring harm.*

ACCOUNTING FOR ME

*Search me, God, and know my heart; test me and
know my anxious thoughts. See if there is any
offensive way in me, and lead me
in the way everlasting.*

—Psalm 139:23–24

Even as the two become one in your marriage, you are still very much individuals. You are different people who might experience the same situation but perceive it differently. You have your own desires, ambitions, gifts, and even flaws. Growing closer to each other doesn't mean you lose your identity or individuality.

For some this is an important reminder, and for others this is freeing. The knitting together of two souls is like two fabrics being woven together to create a masterpiece. Marriage is not about turning into each other but allowing your unique identities to be intertwined together to make something new and profound.

One of the greatest gifts you can give your marriage is to know yourself more. Understanding yourself and maintaining a great sense of self-awareness allows you to bring health and life into your relationship. When you are unaware of your own shortcomings or tendencies, it makes navigating disagreements and daily life challenging for those around you. That's because people who lack self-awareness are often less likely to receive feedback well, and they're more apt to struggle to empathize or understand another person's perspective. They constantly view their own contributions as greater than anyone else's. When self-awareness remains undeveloped, it can lead to frustration and harm within a marriage.

Whether you would describe yourself as generally a self-aware person or not, it's always helpful to grow in this area. The journey of knowing yourself better doesn't come through self-examination; it comes from turning to the one who knows you best: your Creator. Your thoughts of yourself can be deceptive. You need wisdom from outside of yourself. God is the one who created you, knows everything about you, and loves you in spite of your greatest flaws. He is the one who can provide a true reflection of who you are and the areas needing growth.

When David writes Psalm 139, these areas are what he is describing. He understands there are aspects of himself that he is unaware of or areas that he is blind to. So, he asks for God to search his heart and to reveal those areas to him. But he doesn't just stop at asking God to reveal these aspects of his heart to him. He asks for God to lead him in removing these offensive ways from him.

This should be a constant prayer in your marriage. Allowing God to reveal and cleanse you of anything offensive in your hearts will enable you to be better people and spouses. It will give way to a healthier marriage as you ask for God to work within you as individuals.

Let's pray: Lord, please search my heart and reveal to me any areas that are a grievance to you or others. Make me aware of the aspects of me that are not of you, then cleanse me of them. Amen.

WHEN THE EARTH CRUMBLES BENEATH YOU

"Though the mountains be shaken and the hills be removed, yet my unfailing love for you will not be shaken nor my covenant of peace be removed," says the Lord, who has compassion on you.

—Isaiah 54:10

What do you do when you and your spouse are no longer growing together—when, for one reason or another, it seems like your relationship isn't all you expected it would be and you're facing challenges you never thought you would face together? What do you do when the silence between the two of you is deafening? Or when harsh words are the only ones you can muster toward each other? How do you respond when you feel rejected, and intimacy is nowhere to be found?

I think it's safe to say that every married couple, in varying degrees, can relate to the angst and pain of these moments. It could be living in the disparity of disconnection physically, emotionally, or mentally from each other. It might even be a great offense in your marriage, such as dishonesty or disloyalty. You might question whether your marriage can survive its current state or whether or not it can, or even should, endure the blow it's been dealt. Sometimes your relationship may just seem off and you can't figure out what changed, but you know continuing down this path will lead you only further and further away from each other.

The feeling of the ground shaking beneath you is unsettling. If you let it, your mind will take you to plenty of places you should never go. These are the moments when you must lean in to the promises of Jesus and plant your feet firmly on the security you have in him. Before you even begin to think through the next steps for your marriage, you must place all of your hope and assurance in your Savior. There is nothing that can take away the Lord's unfailing love for you. This is a promise he has given you, and it's one you can keep even in the difficult times of your marriage.

The picture being painted in Isaiah 54 is one of great hope and victory. The prophet was given a glimpse of the promise to come in the life of Jesus and, ultimately, in his second return. For the people of God living thousands of years ago, they were eager to see the restoration in their land, for their families, and for their world. We get to see a fuller picture of what Isaiah was describing, because we are living after the death and resurrection of Jesus. You see, this has great eternal implications for your life, but it also has power in your life and marriage today. The love of the Lord for you will never be shaken, and he will have compassion on you even in the most trying times of your marriage.

Let's pray: Jesus, you know every detail of my marriage and every longing of my heart. I'm looking to your love to hold us up when we fall short in ways big and small. Fill me up with your assurance and strength. Even when the ground is shaking beneath me, remind me of your unfailing love and compassion. Amen.

FOSTERING A SPIRIT OF PATIENCE

*Whoever is patient has great understanding, but
one who is quick-tempered displays folly.*

—Proverbs 14:29

I'm known around my house for misplacing important daily items such as my keys and wallet. It doesn't matter how dedicated I am in my mind to placing these things in one spot. They always end up lost.

If there is anyone who can attest to this, it's my husband. This trait of mine makes appearances at the worst of times. It's often during a hectic morning of wrangling the kids to get out the door. One child is having a classic toddler meltdown about wanting his *other* fire truck that is identical to the one in his hand, and the other child just spit up all over his second outfit for the day. The diaper bag is successfully packed, anticipating the many situations that may come our way over the course of the two hours we will be away from home. Dale gets the baby strapped in his car seat, then herds our oldest to the garage. I grab the diaper bag, coffee, water bottle, and any random toys in my path that might prove to be useful during our car ride.

We both arrive at the car, then Dale asks where the keys are. I quickly search my brain for an answer, responding with, "In the diaper bag."

Dale kindly responds with, "I looked, and they're not there."

So, I race back inside the house, still searching my brain, struggling to recall where I placed the car keys. I find them in the pocket of the jacket I wore the day before. I make a mad dash back to the car, where our two lovely children are now screaming, and my husband can only muster up a "I'm mildly frustrated but love you anyways" smile.

I would love to report that misplacing the car keys is a rare occurrence, but it happens far more frequently than I'd like. Are there many ways we could avoid this situation? Yes. I could remember where I put my keys. But explaining how things could be better in the midst of a high-stress situation won't make anything better, and both Dale and I know that. Instead, Dale graciously extends patience for me in moments like this.

It's as Proverbs 14 says: Exercising patience lends itself to a higher degree of understanding, whereas allowing your frustration to get the best of you is unwise. This is a powerful discipline to exercise in your marriage. When either of you allow your anger to drive the situation, things will turn from bad to worse. Refraining from responding to each other in anger, and instead exercising patience, will enable space for the situation to improve.

Your relationship will gain far more ground in difficult situations when both of you choose to show patience rather than anger. This will open the door for discussion on how to make things better instead of shutting down any opportunity for constructive conversation.

Let's pray: Jesus, please help us choose patience over anger so that our marriage is a place of love and kindness toward each other. Amen.

THE HARD CALL OF COMMITMENT

Carry each other's burdens, and in this way you will fulfill the law of Christ.

—Galatians 6:2

Marriage brings out all of the good and bad in each other. This can lead to a great number of wonderful memories and some really difficult ones. The way you and your spouse endure the blunders, missteps, and sin of each other matters. Just about every decision both of you make, and every action you take, will affect each other. The transformation of two becoming one means your shortcomings, bad habits, and temptations directly impact your relationship.

In order to maintain your commitment to each other, you have to learn how to endure the missteps each of you will make. This is hard and painful. When we think of how to actually do this, it's not Galatians 6:2 that comes to mind.

We usually hear the call to bear each other's burdens for those who are needlessly suffering or going through a difficult time. We don't associate this verse as a response to someone's sin, but that's actually the context behind this verse. Just before we get to this verse, we read about a person being caught in sin. Out of this situation follows the need to bear each other's burdens. The Bible cautions us not to fall in sin ourselves as we are helping another through their own sin. But if you can help a fellow believer carry the weight of their own sin, then you ought to.

Carrying the weight of another can feel uncomfortably intimate when it comes to your marriage. If you see the one you love struggling with a certain sin pattern, your role is not to judge or shame but to help carry the load. Recognizing the temptation and struggle of sin in one another is a shared responsibility in marriage. As a couple, you should seek to lovingly bring it into the light and present a willingness to help work through it.

Depending on the situation, bearing burdens in marriage can take on any number of forms. They may look like finding outside help, offering accountability, making space to talk about it free of shame, or even committing to pray together about the specific sin.

It is important to note that this verse does not mean accepting the sin or engaging in codependency. If there is a way for you to walk alongside, support, and care for each other as either one of you works through your sin, then you should do so.

It won't be easy or painless. Supporting each other through your sin will require a lot of selflessness and dependence on the strength of Jesus. In fact, it will be through only your reliance on him that you can do this. This is also not to suggest you must remain in your marriage if the sin of abandonment, abuse, or adultery has been committed against you.

Embracing every aspect of marriage includes the challenges of bearing the burdens of each other.

Let's pray: Jesus, show us how to walk alongside each other in our worst moments. Give us the wisdom to know how to bear each other's burdens. Help us love through our shortcomings and not display judgment or shame. Amen.

DIFFERENT, NOT BETTER OR WORSE

There are different kinds of gifts, but the same Spirit distributes them. There are different kinds of service, but the same Lord. There are different kinds of working, but in all of them and in everyone it is the same God at work.

—1 Corinthians 12:4–6

The early hours of the day are the most productive for Dale. Even he will admit that, as the day progresses, he continues to lose energy. After 2:00 p.m., he's at an all-time low for the day. This means all of his most ambitious objectives for the day are cared for long before lunchtime.

I, on the other hand, am very different. It takes a good cup of coffee and a few hours of being awake for me to even think about being productive for the day. My energy builds as the day goes on, so I'm usually off and running by the time all of Dale's energy has been depleted. On paper these differences don't seem like they could turn into complications.

As my energy kicks in and I'm getting everything checked off the list around the house while he is firmly planted on the couch, I've had to remind myself that Dale works best in the mornings. In my moments of wanting help with certain tasks, I have to remember he's not lazy, inconsiderate, or unhelpful. Dale's already been up and running for several hours by the time I can find enough motivation to get the necessary things done. Instead of him being frustrated that I'm still sleeping while he's up making breakfast, or me feeling that he's inconsiderate while I pick up the toys around his feet as he watches his favorite show, we must be mindful of the way we are different.

The two of us have distinct ways of doing things and varying strengths that don't always line up in our marriage the way we'd like them to. As challenging as it is to keep perspective in these moments, we know it's harmful to our marriage to expect each other to operate the exact same way. This doesn't mean my way, or his way, is better or worse. It means we are different and filled with a variety of gifts and strengths that have been given to us by God.

Paul's words to the church of Corinth in 1 Corinthians 12 reminds us to celebrate our differences before the Lord. The differences of you and your spouse may not seem like gifts when they are opposite of each other, but they are. Instead of wanting to change each other, pray for God to help you celebrate the unique ways you've been created.

Let's put it into practice: When you notice differences between you and your spouse, how can you choose to celebrate them? This might look like verbally complimenting each other or simply remaining silent instead of offering correction. Alternatively, you might tackle a task by dividing the responsibilities, coming up with a due date, and trusting the other to get it done.

BETTER TOGETHER

As iron sharpens iron, so one person sharpens another.

—Proverbs 27:17

There is always a lot of criticism around mindlessly scrolling through social media, but I've actually found a few useful tips during these times. I'm sheepishly admitting to you that social media showed me what the steel rod in my knife block is intended for. I had absolutely no idea that the knife block I received as a wedding gift included a tool to sharpen my knives. Once I discovered this, I quickly searched for videos on exactly how to use it properly. It's such a delight to slice open a watermelon with great ease without throwing my back out in the process. Prior to this knowledge, my knives had reached a place where they were pretty useless to me. It wasn't until I used the steel rod that they became useful again.

This is the same principle illustrated in Proverbs 27:17. Just as iron is used to sharpen another piece of iron, we are in need of other people to sharpen us. As your bond in marriage strengthens, so should your ability to offer growth in each other's lives. It's in the safety of your relationship that each other's sharp and rough edges can be smoothed out.

There are opportunities for growth in your individual lives that God will bring to light through your relationship. God will use the two of you to keep each other accountable, motivated, and encouraged. It's truly amazing how God will use the insights of another person—somebody who sees all of you—in order to make you better. Dale and I have been able to call out certain tendencies or even blind spots in each other in a way no other relationship in our lives has allowed.

God using your marriage to help you grow, stretch, and strengthen is mutually beneficial. Both you and your spouse should be open to corrections from each other. There must be a mutual sense of vulnerability, personal connection, and trust for growth to be accomplished. God will use your relationship to make each other better, when you are willing. You can truly be better together when you let down your guard and allow God to use each other in your life. This is not about one partner towering over the other, or the other being weaker and in need of strengthening. It's about mutual submission to each other and maintaining a posture and dedication to grow.

One of the great beauties of marriage is that God will use the two of you to make each other better.

Let's reflect: Are each of you open to receiving corrections from the other? How do you each respond when the other points out areas of improvement in your life? How can you be more open not only to receive but also to welcome opportunities of growth from your marriage?

BETTER THAN THE MOVIES

How delightful is your love, my sister, my bride! How much more pleasing is your love than wine, and the fragrance of your perfume more than any spice!

—Song of Solomon 4:10

Everyone enjoys a good love story. Even action movies always find a way to sneak in a love angle. It's something many of us can relate to, either through experience or a desire in our heart.

The trouble with movies is they often display a flattened version of love. Hollywood usually shows one stage in a couple's love story as if it lasts forever and never changes or fades. They portray this as the ideal situation, and if your love story alters from this, then you believe your love story is lacking. This is simply not true. To set up one aspect of love as the ideal does harm to so many marriages. The truth is that our love stories can be more complex and, by extension, even more rewarding than they are in the movies.

The Song of Solomon is an ongoing dialogue between two lovers. They have an excitement and a passion for each other. This book is unlike any other book you will read in the Bible, as it describes in great detail the emotional and physical love between this couple. In chapter four, the groom is talking to his bride. He describes how much he delights in her as being better than wine. He has been captivated by her love, and it's about more than merely physical attraction.

What these two lovers share should be our hope in our own marriages. We should desire to truly delight in each other's company and presence. We should want our homes and relationships to be a space of happiness and enjoyment. The excitement of love doesn't have to fade away as the years pass. Your love might vary from season to season, but that can also be a sign that your love is strengthening rather than fading. To still find joy and delight in your spouse when their looks are less than youthful, their job changes, and their dreams evolve is a sign of maturity in your love. Likewise, you should long for your spouse to delight in you.

Making space for laughter and fun in your relationship is important. It becomes easy to be pulled down by the ongoing responsibilities and challenges life throws your way. But we can't let these things pull the life and delight right out of our marriage. These are the moments to lean in to your love for each other more and to see new aspects of each other to delight in. Allow your marriage to captivate your heart day after day.

Let's put it into action: Pick one day this week to learn something new about each other. Think of a way to engage in a conversation or observe a new aspect of your spouse. Allow yourselves to delight in the person you have married.

FORGIVING YOURSELF

Who is a God like you, who pardons sin and forgives the transgression of the remnant of his inheritance? You do not stay angry forever but delight to show mercy.

—Micah 7:18

Good memory is a double-edged sword. It's wonderful to make others feel special by remembering the little things that will go a long way. But it can be a curse for your own overall health. When your brain so kindly replays the unwise decisions you've made or the hurtful words you've uttered, you can begin to view yourself only through the perspective of these situations. If you allow the tragedies of your past to take residence in your mind today, then you might see the effects seeping into your marriage.

I have allowed mistakes from past relationships to convince me I'm not deserving of love in my marriage. Replaying situations from years ago has also caused me to question whether or not I am truly changed, or whether or not I will see these failures creep back into my life or, even worse, my marriage. This way of thinking proved to be harmful to my relationship. I would find myself withdrawing from my husband in hopes of not repeating the past. Unfortunately, our obsession to correct mistakes from our past can lead to new hurts.

Part of moving forward requires taking the necessary steps to correct sin, but it has to be met with forgiveness. You restrict the freedom Jesus gives you when you remain captive to the memory of former sins. This is the wisdom the prophet Micah speaks over the nation of Israel. During the time of Micah's prophecy, Israel and Judah are on the verge of imploding from the failures of their leaders. Micah speaks words of judgment over them, but they are accompanied by a beautiful promise of restoration. Israel and Judah had a checkered past and they weren't exactly on an upward trend during the life of Micah, but he still tells them God will pardon their sin. Not only will he forgive them for every single blunder ever committed, but he also delights in showing them mercy.

Of course, those specific words were not written to you and me. They were written to the people of Judah and Israel. Yet we can understand God's same heart of forgiveness and delight in showing mercy to be our promise. This is most fully seen in the life and death of Jesus.

You are already fully pardoned for every transgression ever committed and even more because of Jesus. Jesus delights in showing you mercy. This is your state before the living God. It should also be the way you view yourself: forgiven and shown mercy. When you extend forgiveness and mercy to yourself, the way you interact in your marriage will change. This allows you to be in a healthier place to give and receive love in your marriage.

Let's reflect: In what areas are you harboring unforgiveness about yourself? Can you see how these areas might be impacting your relationship? What would it look like to take a step toward forgiving yourself and extending mercy?

SURRENDER YOUR MARRIAGE

I have been crucified with Christ and I no longer live, but Christ lives in me. The life I now live in the body, I live by faith in the Son of God, who loved me and gave himself for me.

—Galatians 2:20

I'm sure you don't need me to tell you that you are unable to control life. It's probably something you realized a long time ago, and it wasn't due to lack of trying. There is an unrealistic sense of security we have when we think we can control a situation. This is even the case for marriage. To some degree, we have a disillusioned sense of control because, after all, we chose to marry the person we've married. Even if your spouse continues to be exactly who you've known and expected them to be, your marriage doesn't exist in a vacuum. There are many other outside factors that impact your marriage. Things like jobs, children, health issues, financial troubles, or any number of curveballs thrown your way quickly remind you that you are not in control.

There is an aspect of your marriage that must be surrendered to God. You will find yourself in a lot of pain if you are constantly trying to mold or move your marriage in the way you want it to be. There are a lot of reasons this will lead you to heartache, but one of the main ones is that we don't like it when our spouse tries to control us. Marriage is a partnership and not about finding ways to change each other. I once had a friend describe her life philosophy as one of leaning in to an ongoing willingness to be available, flexible, and even surprised by God. There is so much wisdom in living this way.

She's tapped into a mentality of surrender that God has called all of us to. Yes, even our marriages should be lived in surrender to the one who can actually control all things. When Paul describes our state of life in Christ, he says it's one of change and that it's not really our own. Before Jesus, we all lived with our self-interests as the central focus, but that was all changed at the point of salvation. Our old ways of thinking and living are gone. With each passing day, the old you continues to vanish. Jesus is the one guiding you and leading you. The act of surrender is ongoing and should permeate every aspect of your life.

Jesus wants you to surrender your marriage to him. He wants you to give your worries to him. You can trust that his plans for your relationship, future, and life are far better than what you have in mind. Instead of fighting for control, it's time to lay it at the feet of Jesus.

Let's reflect: Which area or areas of your marriage are you trying to control? Perhaps it's certain characteristics in your spouse, or it could be you laying out the plans and dreams of your lives together, or maybe it's your way of doing things being the core of your household. How can you surrender aspects of your marriage to Jesus?

COMMITTED TO BUILDING

The wise woman builds her house, but with her
own hands the foolish one tears hers down.

—Proverbs 14:1

There's something about a small human impersonating you that makes you realize how powerful your influence really is. My toddler has been a mirror into my subconscious. His reactions to situations or phrases he utters are a replica of who I am. He's displayed aspects of me that I never realized existed. This experience has been life altering for me and required me to exercise a greater sense of self-awareness.

As wives, we influence our families in many ways. You might not always see it, but you influence your spouse, just as they do you. The Bible is clear that you both have great influence in your household. For the sake of the health and growth of your family, it's vital that you both are mindful and intentional with your influence.

For example, if you had a terrible day at work and you allow that frustration to lead your interactions once you get home, it will likely cause a domino effect of reactions. It can be hard to end the cycle of reactions, but at some point you must. It's the little decisions in the day-to-day that you must actively choose to build up and not tear down.

This week's proverb is using the metaphor of building your house to refer to your entire life. It takes effort and mindfulness to build up your house. You have to actively choose words that will build up your relationships and not tear them down. It takes effort not to allow your frustrations at work to become your frustrations at home. Being mindful of the way your habits impact those around you and your marriage embodies the wise woman choosing to build her home.

To be clear, the verse is not referring to building and keeping an orderly house in a literal sense, but rather is calling you to keep your eyes open to the way you impact others. Choose to let your words, tone, habits, and actions build up the people around you and not tear them down.

Being mindful of the way you treat others is a call to every Christian. Let your love for others exemplify your faith in Jesus and the way he has transformed your life.

As you move through your week, recite the following prayer over the people in your life to build on the words of Proverbs 14:1.

Let's pray: Lord, give me eyes to see the influence you've given me over my house. Let my hands be used to build up and not tear down. When this task feels too heavy, let me look to you. Amen.

FAITHFULNESS

Let love and faithfulness never leave you;
bind them around your neck, write them on the
tablet of your heart.

—Proverbs 3:3

I often tell my husband how happy I am to be past the dating phase of life. There was a sense of uncertainty that came with dating that I didn't enjoy. Dating couples can easily decide, for any reason, that they just don't want to be in that relationship anymore. It's not always a mutual agreement, and that's the part that made me so nervous.

As you move from dating to marriage, the commitment level changes dramatically. The great hope is that a sense of security and ongoing commitment should be a pillar in your relationship. Throughout the trials and tribulations of your marriage, you know that both of you remain committed.

Your loyalty and trust in each other should bring a deep sense of security and assurance. When commitment is lost, there is great pain and damage to the relationship. This is not to say God is unable to bring redemption and restoration in miraculous ways, but rather the road to healing can be long and hard. There should be no shame or guilt if you've been in a relationship where commitment was lost. The hope is that, in your current relationship, both partners maintain a high sense of commitment to each other. It doesn't matter how bad your habits are or the many ways you will change throughout your lifetime because marriage is an ongoing commitment. In order for this to be a reality in your marriage, you have to live out the wisdom of Proverbs 3:3.

Solomon lays out two important attributes that we should have in our lives: love and faithfulness. The Hebrew word for love in this verse is *hesed*, which is always used to describe God's love for his people. It's a very difficult word to translate into English because of how rich and deep the meaning is. Oftentimes, it's translated as "loving kindness" because it is so much greater than an emotional love. It's a type of love that demands kindness, gentleness, mercy, loyalty, and faithfulness all in one. We are to model this same kind of love and faithfulness to others, as God has done for us.

Living out this verse about faithfulness is not limited to never having an affair. Being faithful and loving to each other is about showing kindness, gentleness, mercy, and loyalty. It's about constantly being reliable in your marriage. Your spouse should know they can count on you to root them on when life is hard. You should know you can count on their to support you when your decision doesn't go as planned. You should encourage each other when you fail, and call out the good when you see it. It's about standing by each other's side and being a person you can each depend on in every way.

Let's pray: Heavenly Father, thank you for your steadfast love. Show us how to love each other in the way you have loved us. Grant us the courage to support each other when we fail, and lift each other up when we do well. When we feel discouraged in this pursuit, remind us of the love you've shown us. Amen.

YOUR PROVIDER

And my God will meet all your needs according to
the riches of his glory in Christ Jesus.

—Philippians 4:19

Figuring out what it looks like to provide and be provided for within the confines of marriage is important. For some couples, one person may be depended on as the breadwinner. For others, it might be more of a discussion of what it looks like to be provided for emotionally and mentally. I truly believe the expectation and mutual understanding of what should be provided by each spouse can change from marriage to marriage and even from season to season. What may be incredibly important to one couple might not even be on another couple's radar. But for all marriages, it's pressing for both sides to agree and make known what each expects for the other to provide.

When Dale and I were first married, our health insurance was provided through my employer. It was actually a huge blessing for Dale, because his employer didn't offer this as a benefit. This became a concern as I considered other employment opportunities. There was a great sense of pressure for me to select only a job that would continue to provide the same types of benefits. At one point, I was being considered for a position I was incredibly excited about. It was for a cause that was very close to my heart, but it didn't offer the same types of benefits. I felt sad about the thought of rejecting this opportunity because of our personal needs. In this season of life, I was needed to provide health insurance for my family, yet I felt a great weight at having to walk away from something I deeply desired in order to deliver the benefits we needed.

There are many areas in your own marriage that need to be provided for, whether by you or your spouse. Sometimes, it might seem as if areas that should be provided are not, and you don't know how to respond. There may also be a scenario in which something that was once provided by the other no longer is. In these situations, it's important to turn to your Ultimate Provider. God promises to provide for all of your needs. That may be directly through your spouse, a realignment in your relationship, or even through you. God is not short on resources or ways to provide for the things you need. Remember that not everything you *want* will be provided for, but everything you *need* will be.

So, whether you have practical or relational needs that are not being provided for, bring them before your Provider. He hears the cries of your heart and answers. Hold tightly to the promises given to all believers in Philippians that God will care for your needs.

Let's pray: Jesus, I trust you with every area of my life. I trust that you will provide for every need of my family. Please, help us turn to you and remember that you are our Ultimate Provider. Amen.

HONORING AFFECTION

*Let the husband render to his wife the affection due
her, and likewise also the wife to her husband.*

—1 Corinthians 7:3, NKJV

It doesn't come as naturally to talk about sex as it does to do
it. Yet it's a leading issue in many marriages. A lack of intimacy is
more than a lack of physical affection. It can take on many other
shapes and forms. Physical intimacy may not be an issue, but
you may find emotional intimacy is lacking. When a marriage has
a lack of intimacy in any form, it means there is an aspect of the
relationship that is not as open, vulnerable, or safe as it should
be. It's hard to be vulnerable in every aspect of your life with one
person, but that is what marriage should be. The connection God
designed between you both is all-encompassing.

Paul's words to the church of Corinth show us how important it is to engage in intimacy within marriage. Many translations
render the Greek word *opheilé* as "duty or obligation." This is
not an incorrect translation. It's actually very literal. It's hard for
a culture like ours not to misunderstand this verse as cold and
harsh, because it uses the word duty in relation to marriage. We
don't like the idea of seeing any aspect of our marriage as an
obligation or a duty; it sounds as if it's void of love or choice. This
is quite the opposite of what is being expressed in this verse.

The biblical understanding of marriage is that it is a covenant
between two people. There are promises made to care for each
other, and there are many ways in which that fleshes itself out
in real life. One of the ways to truly care for each other in marriage is to commit to intimacy. Yes, physical intimacy is part of
that, but so is emotional and spiritual intimacy. There is a mutual

understanding within marriage that you will care for each other in these ways—and, in fact, there is a sense of obligation to these things. The topic of intimacy in all its forms shouldn't make us uncomfortable or be labeled as "dirty." God created us to experience intimacy in all its forms, including sexual intimacy. We should not feel a sense of shame or guilt for desiring to be intimate with each other in marriage. God intended for you and your spouse to long for intimacy with each other. Through intimacy, there is a knitting together and bonding that grows stronger and stronger as you both remain committed to each other.

Being affectionate and intimate within marriage won't always come easy, but choosing to work through that together is being true to the promises you've made to each other.

Let's reflect: In a quiet place where it's just you and your spouse, reflect on the following questions: Are there areas of intimacy that are lacking in your marriage? Is this something you both have simply learned how to live with, or are you trying to work through it? What would it look like for you to stay true to your promise of intimacy with each other?

THE SAME TEAM

Jesus knew their thoughts and said to them,
"Every kingdom divided against itself will be
ruined, and every city or household divided against
itself will not stand."

—Matthew 12:25

I was on the cheer team in high school and, as you can imagine, there was a lot of drama. My freshman year could have made a great reality show. Our team was filled with girls whose only similarity was being in cheer. I don't think a more diverse and mixed group of girls could have existed. The amount of tension between all of the girls became a major problem when it came to succeeding as a team.

A large part of cheerleading requires trust and respect for your teammates, especially if you are the flier, the person being thrown in the air. The flier has to be able to trust that the stunt team will catch her and keep her safety at the forefront of their minds. If this trust is not in place, then the team is unsuccessful. It doesn't matter how talented and gifted the individuals on the team are—if they can't work together, then they fail. This is exactly what happened for most of my freshman year. We didn't operate as a team but as individuals.

It took my entire freshman year for us to understand our division was leading to our failure. It wasn't until we respected and treated one another as teammates that we became a decent cheer team. The lesson of teamwork is not only important for sports teams but also in much of life, especially marriage.

In Matthew 12, Jesus reminds the religious leaders about this truth. The religious leaders question whether Jesus is truly the promised Messiah or if he is operating out of allegiance to Satan. Jesus quickly settles this dispute by sharing the simple principle that "a household divided against itself will not stand." He shines a spotlight on how ridiculous it would be for Satan to drive out his own demons, for that would be working against himself.

The ageless "a house divided will fall" principle is perfectly applicable to marriage. When spouses choose to see each other as the enemy, or actively work against each other, their relationship will be negatively impacted. There is no way to see your love, compassion, and commitment to each other grow if you're working against the other. It's critical for you both to always remember you are on the same team, a tag team. When one of you wins, you both win. When one of you loses, you both lose.

You must vow to always see each other as a fellow teammate and never as the enemy. This will set yourself up to maintain a marriage that will last. There will be moments when it's hard to keep this vow, but staying true to each other in this way will impact your marriage for the better. Vowing to be friends over enemies, regardless of what life throws at you, will bring you only closer together.

Let's pray: Lord, will you guard our hearts against seeing each other as the enemy? Help us value and cherish each other in a way that will always lead us closer together rather than apart. Help us strive to be a house that never divides and to remember we are always on the same team. Amen.

A DEVOTED HEART

As Solomon grew old, his wives turned his heart
after other gods, and his heart was not fully devoted
to the Lord his God, as the heart of David
his father had been.

—1 Kings 11:4

Solomon was the richest and smartest man in the known world at the time. But as the king of Israel, Solomon had an unsanctioned number of wives and concubines. As commonplace as this was for kings, this was not the way God wanted his people to live. He had actually spoken against this way of life over and over again. Solomon took on many wives as a way to build safety and security with neighboring nations. He was really trying to strategize and plan ways to ensure his kingdom would last. Ultimately, this had a great impact on the faith, heart, and reign of Solomon.

Apart from the fact that God never intended for a man to have more than one wife, the wives Solomon did have often pressured him to compromise his faith. They came from nations that worshipped other gods and, over the course of time, Solomon began to worship them, too. He turned away from the faith he had known since a young age. As he began to shift away from his faith in God, he began to lead differently. There was a parallel line between Solomon's change in faith and his leadership. As one took a turn for the worse, so did the other. After his death, the kingdom of Israel divided into two separate nations. Solomon allowed his wives to lead him further and further away from God.

As a couple, your opinions, passions, and thoughts impact each other deeply. The way you view the world and the people around you will alter the way your spouse sees the world. The way they understand life issues will have a significant impact on you. This isn't a bad thing. In fact, that's exactly the way God intended it to be. Marriage is all about two people becoming one.

It's important in your relationship that you be intentional about pointing each other closer to God. Let each other see the way you depend on the Lord. How you lean on Jesus when life becomes too hard.

It's not about being the perfect Christian but about watching each other depend on Jesus. Your spouse's faith can be strengthened as they watch your faith grow. Your faith can be encouraged as you watch their daily relationship with Jesus.

Let's reflect: Do you allow your spouse to see the depths of your faith? Do you share your deepest prayers with one another? How can you give each other a greater glimpse into your faith?

OPEN TO CORRECTION

Mockers resent correction, so they avoid the wise.

—Proverbs 15:12

I have always dreaded employee reviews. It's never easy to sit in your manager's office, knowing their objective is to evaluate your performance for the year. A good manager will equally share the positive aspects of your performance, but there are always a few areas that need improvement. I was actually once told in a review that I need to work on receiving corrections better. As you can imagine, that was painful to hear. For me, it was a hit to my pride, because I would love to hear there are no areas of improvement needed. It was also a realization that in order to grow, I needed to be able to accept constructive criticism.

To be sure, not every critique is constructive. It takes discernment to know what to apply and what to throw away. This is truly a critical aspect of becoming more like the person God created us to be. We shouldn't be like the person described in this proverb. Our hope should be the opposite. We should welcome correction and let wisdom be spoken in our lives.

One of the best relationships to apply this wisdom to is your marriage. The person who sees you day in and day out is your spouse. They get to witness your reaction, habit, and response to just about every situation. They are privy to your raw emotion and less-than-professional response.

It takes a mature person not only to receive corrections but also to welcome them. And within your marriage, both of you should welcome corrections from each other. Certainly, feedback should be given in a loving and mindful manner as part of your marriage. Your spouse should feel comfortable bringing to light ways you've hurt them. You should feel comfortable bringing up ways they have hurt you. When correction is welcomed between the two of you, there is opportunity for growth. It also allows you to learn how to love each other better.

The delivery of the correction is just as important as the critique itself. It will take practice to learn how to share this feedback lovingly with each other. It requires a sense of tenderness and respect for each other. Correction should never be used as a weapon but as a way to engage further in your relationship. As uncomfortable as it may be, creating a common space for loving correction will help you grow closer together.

Let's pray: Heavenly Father, let our marriage be a place of growth and maturity. Help us welcome corrections and learn how to share them lovingly. I want us to hear about our blind spots and shortcomings from each other, where it's safe and free of judgment. Amen.

CALLING EACH OTHER FRIEND

Walk with the wise and become wise, for a companion of fools suffers harm.

—Proverbs 13:20

I recently decided to unfollow social media accounts that constantly post negative content about spouses, even though they claim to be marriage accounts. I'm certainly not against honest and open conversations about the difficulties of marriage, as these types of conversations have served to remind me that I'm not alone in some of my struggles. It's nice to be seen, to be heard, and to know your experience is common. I had originally followed certain social media accounts as a newlywed for these reasons, but I soon realized they were doing more harm than good.

To constantly be reminded of the challenges, difficulties, and annoyances in marriage is far from helpful. In fact, I found it was damaging to my perception of my marriage. Couples begin to adopt tunnel vision of their marriage when they are flooded with criticism and negativity in relation to marriage. This perception takes a deeper root in your marriage when these are the types of conversations you are having with your friend groups, coworkers, and acquaintances.

When you surround yourself with people who have a negative view of their spouse, it won't be long before you, too, will have a critical view of your own marriage. What begins as a simple, harmless, and even great sense of camaraderie can end in hurt toward your relationship.

In Proverbs 13, we are reminded of the importance of who we surround ourselves with. If you befriend other couples who are trying to grow in their marriage, you will have a desire to do the same. If the people you surround yourself with are filled with negativity and animosity about their marriage, you will begin to be jaded about your own marriage. Out of this negative perception of your spouse will come harm, as you will see only the things you wish were different.

It is important to be aware of how your friend group is impacting your marriage. This doesn't mean you necessarily have to stop being friends with people who are negative or critical. But seeking and maintaining friendships that encourage you to love your spouse and grow in your marriage is crucial. You will find the healthy habits of other couples inspiring and something you will want to see transpire in your own relationship. Friends desiring to honor, value, and love their spouse as Jesus has called them will help your own marriage reflect these same attributes.

Let's reflect: *Are there friends in your life whose critical comments of their marriage outweigh the good? Do you see yourself engaging in similar conversations about your own relationship when you are around them? Can you think of one friend who is intentional about loving and valuing their spouse? In what ways can you develop this friendship further?*

DEALING WITH CONFLICT

*Consider it pure joy, my brothers and sisters,
whenever you face trials of many kinds, because
you know that the testing of your faith
produces perseverance.*

—James 1:2–3

Engaging in personal conflict is never exciting. As I look back on my upbringing, I would say my family held to the "sweeping it under the rug" method of dealing with conflict. We didn't like to bring up hurts, offenses, or disagreements from one another, so we would push them away and hope they would resolve themselves. Sometimes the passing of time would help certain situations, but most conflicts remained unresolved and snowballed into far larger situations. In my marriage I've had to be actively aware of this tendency and fight against it.

Addressing conflict is not a healthy skill either Dale or I brought into our marriage. It is something we've had to practice and learn within our relationship. It's not always comfortable, but it is beneficial. In this process, we've learned how to communicate with each other better. Part of that has included how we bring up our hurts or offenses and even when to bring them up. Timing and tone are important.

Taking the steps not only to address conflict within your relationship but also to know how to go about it with your spouse is crucial. The opening of James talks about how Christians should deal with trials in their lives. His instructions can equally be applied to marriage.

God promises to use trials of various kinds, including conflict. This doesn't mean God places trials and conflict in your life to teach you a lesson. It means we live in a world where these things are inevitable, but God will use them for a greater purpose. The hurt and pain you come across doesn't have to be wasted. It can be used to strengthen your faith and build perseverance. This is true in your marriage.

When you both commit to dealing with your conflict, you will strengthen your bond. It may not feel that way as you're talking about it, but with each conversation and open line of communication, you can chip away at the things that drive you apart. Sharing ways you have hurt each other allows for the opportunity of correction. Hearing about the ways you've offended each other gives you the chance to see things from a different perspective. When you have an agreed expectation and shared effort to address conflict, the roots of your relationship will grow deeper.

It will be a journey to learn what works best for your relationship, but choosing to invest in this area will always be beneficial. As scary and uncertain as this might seem, you can take comfort in knowing you don't have to do it alone. God will use your conflict for the strength and growth of your marriage.

Let's put it into practice: Make time to have a conversation about how you handle conflict in your relationship. Ask each other the hard questions. Do we have a healthy way of dealing with our conflict? In what ways can we improve our willingness to communicate when we are offended, hurt, or frustrated with each other? Now, commit to each other that this is an area you want to grow in.

THE POWER OF HABIT

"But let the one who boasts boast about this: that they have the understanding to know me, that I am the Lord, who exercises kindness, justice and righteousness on earth, for in these I delight," declares the Lord.

—Jeremiah 9:24

When Jeremiah prophesied to the people of Israel, he was exhorting them about how they should live. The things that should be a central focus in their minds, hearts, and actions are succinctly explained in this verse. Everything we do in life should move us closer toward understanding God more, and exercising kindness, justice, and righteousness toward others. More specifically, the daily habits we establish in our lives should always move us closer to understanding what God wants and draw us closer to him. The subconscious acts we carry out regularly are a window into our hearts.

Living a life as instructed by this week's verse does not happen passively. To have a heart centered on the things God's heart is centered on requires us to be intentional about seeing these things cultivated in our lives. It's through daily habits that you can see kindness, justice, and righteousness be part of the air you breathe.

In the first few years of marriage, my husband and I learned a lot about each other. When we first moved in together, we didn't fully understand how profound the process of learning about each other would be. We had to learn how to adjust to creating a shared home, which meant creating new habits to care for each other well. Dale and I had to learn how to pause when we are upset and evaluate if our frustration is unfair toward each other. I've had to learn not to blurt out the first thoughts in my mind but to reflect on how to phrase my words in a kinder and softer way.

It became so important for us to adjust our personal habits for the betterment of our marriage. Once something becomes a habit in our lives, we no longer think about it. We've repeated it so many times that it becomes subconscious. Some of our habits are healthy and life-giving, whereas others are unhealthy and become hard to correct. There are various types of habits we bring into our relationship, but we should be mindful of the spiritual, physical, and emotional habits that have a large impact.

We should hope for our heart to reflect the heart of God in our marriage. This means the habits we allow to take up residence in our life should uphold the appeal found in Jeremiah 9. It's nearly impossible to separate your marriage from your life, and that's the way God intended it. As you continue to seek a God-centered marriage, be mindful of the habits you allow into your life that will impact your marriage. These habits should lead you to know and understand God more. They should also lead you to show kindness, justice, and righteousness to others—including to each other.

Let's reflect: Over the next week, I encourage you to take an inventory of the habits in your marriage. Which habits lead you to the life described in this week's verse? Which habits do you need to adjust or remove, and why or why not?

AS ONE

*I have given them the glory that you gave me, that
they may be one as we are one—I in them and you
in me—so that they may be brought to complete
unity. Then the world will know that you sent me
and have loved them even as you have loved me.*

—John 17:22–23

One of the most powerful visual images I've seen of what unity looks like in marriage is the unity sand ceremony performed at weddings. As the couple pours the sand out of their own vessel into a shared vessel, the two colors blend and layer unevenly. There is even a point in the process when you can't distinguish the two colors, as they've made a new color all together. There are sections in the new vessel with very apparent separations between the two colors, but it's not an equal representation throughout.

The areas of equal and unequal sand colors are much like marriage. Unity within marriage is the mixing and blending of two people. At times there will be clear distinctions between the two, and at others the blending of lives will be impossible to separate. When a couple is unified, they begin moving in the same direction, supporting each other, and working together for the benefit of each other. Unity doesn't mean completely losing who you are as individuals. It means bringing your individuality and intertwining both together. This is what Jesus wants for all of his people. In John's letter, he describes Christ's desire for all of his people to be unified. This is equally true when it comes to your marriage.

Jesus wants you to be intertwined in your marriage as you are connected to him. He means this in a very spiritual sense, but it's also in the whole of your lives that exists on this side of eternity. When partners are looking to work alongside each other, both of you win. It's not that you have to look out for your best interests, because your spouse is doing that. You are thinking of them and they are thinking of you. This is a far better way to allow your individual identities to be maintained while still joining together as one. The idea of putting the interest of your spouse and marriage above all else shouldn't mean a loss for you. In fact, it means a gain because you are both placing the interests of the other before your own.

Working toward unity in your marriage will allow your relationship to be everything God desires for you, while showing his love to those around you.

Let's pray: Heavenly Father, bring us closer together in marriage. Allow us to desire and work toward unity with each other above all other things. When the fear of losing our own identity rises, remind us that unity doesn't have to be at the expense of ourselves. Amen.

FINANCIAL HEALTH

"No one can serve two masters. Either you will hate the one and love the other, or you will be devoted to the one and despise the other. You cannot serve both God and money."

—Matthew 6:24

Money. It is one of those difficult topics in life and in marriage. It's hard enough to establish a healthy relationship with money on your own, but that challenge is amplified when you add another person to the mix. Agreeing on how much is needed, how much to save, and what to spend it on or save it for is hard work. If these things are not agreed upon, ongoing tension and conflict within your relationship will soon follow.

There is great wisdom in having an established strategy for how to handle your finances, but you must have an understanding before getting to that point. The Bible actually has a lot to say about money. As much as we know money isn't everything, it is nearly impossible to live without it. We live in a world in which money rules, so it would be foolish to live as if money has no significance in your life. In the Gospel written by Matthew, we read the very words of Jesus. His view on money is that you can't serve both money and God. But he doesn't say money is meaningless, only that you can't serve it.

So, what does this mean? It means we have to put money in its rightful place. Money is a resource to be used and stewarded by God, but it is not a god in our lives. The pursuit of making more money and the other temptations that come along with it, like materialism and misplaced happiness, shouldn't be part of the

Christian life. It is our pursuit of God that should be the greater priority and focus within our lives. This should be a relational view and not an individual view. Nothing should take priority in our life over the pursuit of God.

If one partner is constantly chasing a dream of making more money, it will create tension in your marriage. The pursuit will always leave them wanting more, because they will never feel as if they have enough. Neither of you will ever be truly satisfied. Therefore, both of your devotion to strengthening your connection with God must take priority over your effort to amass more money. Both of your hearts and minds should be motivated by your love for Jesus and not material things.

Jesus will never forsake you. He is for the health and life of your marriage. Money has no interest in these things. Maintaining a healthy relationship means recognizing that money is not what will bring happiness and clarity, and that Jesus must remain in the forefront of your relationship at all times. True financial health begins with keeping money in its rightful place and Jesus in his.

Let's reflect: Why might you feel it is important for you both to make more money? How is drawing closer to Jesus more or less important than that? Plan a conversation to assess your view of money as a couple and the ways in which focusing on your devotion to God will help strengthen your bond with each other.

QUALITY OVER QUANTITY

Teach us to number our days, that we may gain a heart of wisdom.

—Psalm 90:12

I wouldn't describe myself as someone who cries easily, especially not during a movie. But there was a movie recently that had me weeping. The opening scene was a couple putting together the nursery for their little girl. There was so much excitement as the couple talked about how the dynamics of their house would change with their newest family member. They were anxious, overwhelmed, and giddy about the future. The next scene was the couple rushing to the hospital for the birth of their baby. Suddenly, the music became really somber as the doctors explained the mother didn't make it. The movie went silent as the dad wept on the floor. I could no longer see past my own tears. I physically felt a weight in the bottom of my stomach as I imagined my life without my husband.

I never finished watching the movie, because it was far too difficult for me to see the grief and pain. As much as we know that no one is promised tomorrow, it's easy to forget. We continue to plan and live like we have a great number of years left together. It's certainly not helpful to live in a sense of fear and never expect tomorrow to arrive. But I think we all too often swing to the other end and become careless or unintentional with our days.

The psalmist reminds us that our days are numbered and that we would be wise to live with that truth in mind.

We have to be cautious about just trying to get through the day, the week, the year, or the decade without ever enjoying the present moments. Stopping to have quality moments with each other is important. It's not about how many days you have spent in the same space, but about how well you occupied that space together. It becomes so easy for couples to live in the practical routine of life without truly enjoying each other's presence. There are many practical benefits to marriage, such as having an extra set of hands around the house or having someone to share the load of life with. But there are more important aspects of marriage that bring joy and happiness, like having someone to share your heart, hopes, and dreams with. One of the greatest joys we can experience in marriage is to be fully known and accepted by our spouse. This is even greater than the practical benefits of marriage.

Becoming so used to tomorrow that you forget to see and hear each other today is painful. Even if you have eighty years left together, you will want to truly spend it together and not merely exist in the same space. Being present for each other will look different from season to season in your marriage, but don't let the expectation of tomorrow rob you of today.

Let's pray: Lord, I don't want to become so occupied with tomorrow that I forget about today. Let us find ways to be present for each other every day. Let us never stop finding joy in the other or take for granted the moments we have together. Amen.

FILLED WITH JOY

May the God of hope fill you with all joy and peace as you trust in him, so that you may overflow with hope by the power of the Holy Spirit.

—Romans 15:13

Have you ever been around someone whose negativity, critical comments, or lack of interest has immediately changed the mood of the room? A person's lack of joy has a way of affecting those around them. This is especially true in marriage.

The mood of one affecting the entire house has happened firsthand in my own relationship. There have been days when either Dale or I seem to suck the joy and excitement right out of our house. It could be because of any number of factors, but we both know exactly when it's happening. We usually try to be relatively lighthearted with each other and our children. One of our favorite family activities is to dance in the kitchen. Dale and I have always enjoyed this, and our boys have adopted the same love.

The songs we dance to have changed dramatically through-out the years. The latest hits now include "Baby Shark" and "Wheels on the Bus." Those light and happy moments are some of the ones we cherish the most, so it's always unfortunate when either of us allows our stress, frustration, or irritability to prevent us from joining in on the fun, or if we become annoyed by the tenth request for "Baby Shark."

Bad days happen, and there should be space for everyone not to be overwhelmed with joy all of the time. But the days filled with joy should be the norm in our marriages rather than the exception. The call for Christians to be filled with joy is common in Scripture. We read similar words as those in the closing of Paul's letter to the Romans. He speaks a blessing of joy and peace over their lives. This is not dependent upon their circumstances but motivated by their trust in God. Paul wants them to be filled with the joy of Jesus because they know their trust can be placed in him.

We often become stealers of joy when we can't put our trust in God to care for us. If we are overwhelmed with unfavorable situations we can't control, we enable those things to take the lead rather than allowing the joy of Jesus to take over. As a couple, be committed to bringing joy into your house and relationship. Be understanding of bad days, but release them to the One who can truly care for them. Allow your trust to be placed in Jesus. Let him replace your worry and frustration for joy and peace. You will be surprised with how contagious your joy will be for each other and the other members of your family.

Let's put it into practice: Think about how you've been around the house lately. How do you bring joy into your relationship? It might look like praying through a situation weighing you down. It might even look like engaging in something fun with each other. Create a plan of ways you can bring and maintain joy in your relationship this week.

ALIGNED MINDSET

*In your relationships with one another, have the
same mindset as Christ Jesus.*

—Philippians 2:5

The trend of manifesting your own outcomes is on the rise. It's the idea that you can consciously attract anything you long for in your life. This can cover a wide range of desires from money to love. If you set your mind to it, then you can see it come to pass. This idea is really tapping into the power of the mind and what can be accomplished if you simply shift your mindset.

Now, this type of thinking goes against what we are told in Scripture. But there is a nugget of truth that we can hold on to: Your mindset matters. What we allow to shape and mold our worldview dictates how we live. Our mindset tells us how to interact with the people around us. Paul knows this is true, and he reminds Christians to have the same mindset as Jesus, to value others above yourself. This is what Jesus modeled. When we align our mindset with Jesus, everything changes. Instead of operating from a place of pride, we start with humility.

A mindset shift from our natural tendencies to what Jesus desires for us includes trading a critical spirit for extending grace or swapping forgiveness for unforgiveness. It's far less about what we are capable of doing and more about the ways the Holy Spirit can shape our mind, heart, and soul like Jesus.

In your marriage, your mindset will align as you both desire to align with Jesus. You will find you grow closer together as you strive to be more like Jesus. Even as your perspective, thinking, and view changes or matures with the passing of time, it's the desire to stay aligned with the heart of Jesus that will keep you aligned as a couple. It is natural for you both to change with age and life experience, but that doesn't mean you have to evolve in a way that drives you apart. You will find you grow closer together as you pursue the life Jesus modeled, to care about each other over yourself.

I've seen this happen in my own marriage. There are certain theological, political, or philosophical views that Dale and I once held on to that we no longer do. It's healthy to grow in the way you think through situations around you, but it must be within the parameters of what Jesus has said. Your relationship should feel the freedom to change and grow in your worldview without fear that you won't recognize who you married. The best way to ensure you won't grow so far apart in these areas is by remaining aligned in your mindset to pursue Jesus.

Let's pray: Jesus, as we continue to grow and change as individuals, may we never stray from our foundation in you. Help us stay true to our commitment to you above all other things and then our commitment to each other. We want for your wisdom and truth to be the greatest influence in every season of our lives. Amen.

LOOSEN YOUR GRIP ON THE FUTURE

Many are the plans in a person's heart, but it is the Lord's purpose that prevails.

—Proverbs 19:21

Dale and I packed an overnight bag, jumped in the car, and drove with no idea where we would be staying for the night. We ended up in Sedona, then made our way over to the Grand Canyon. To this day, it is one of my most cherished memories. We had just found out I was pregnant with our first child, so we spent the entire trip talking about how our lives would change. We dreamed of things we desired to do as our family grew, and we talked about the kind of family we wanted together. We wanted trips just like this one to be a large part of our life together.

Little did we know, spontaneous trips with minimal packing would become a major challenge with babies. That is only one example of how our plans or expectations for the future needed to adjust. It wasn't in our plans to have two children within two and a half years. It wasn't our plan for Dale to completely change careers. It wasn't our plan to find a new church and create all new relationships. It wasn't in our plan for my transition to mother-hood to be accompanied by depression. The list of things that were never in the plan can go on and on.

I'm sure you can write your own list of events that were not in the plan. It's okay to mourn the loss of what you thought would be. It's okay to ask God why and to cry out to him with your pain. Some changed plans are easier to adjust to, whereas others can be devastating. God has never asked you to just move on and pretend everything is okay. He wants you to continue to share your hurt and pain with him in prayer. You can trust that he will bring healing. It may be through other people or through a repositioning of your heart—or any other number of ways—but you can trust he will care for you.

Proverbs 19:21 is a wonderful reminder to keep our futures in perspective. Seeking God in our marriage means holding our futures loosely. There is nothing wrong with dreaming as a couple and even setting goals to work toward, but it's best to keep a loose grip on these things. Desiring the plans of God to prevail over your own will make it easier to deal with the change in plans. It will also allow you to see that his plans are greater than even your best-laid plans.

As a couple, you can trust that God's plans are not to bring harm or punishment. They are for your good. I encourage you to have your hearts set that his will prevails over even your best-laid plans. The plans of the Lord will never fail you.

Let's pray: Father, let our hearts be motivated by your plans. Prepare us for when it seems like our plans have failed, and help us remember your plans have not. I want our future to be led by you and for us to never stop trusting that you will care for us in every way. Amen.

REJOICING AND MOURNING TOGETHER

Rejoice with those who rejoice; mourn with those who mourn.

—Romans 12:15

I placed my one-month-old baby in his crib and climbed into bed with a heavy heart, knowing I had just seen my grandpa for the last time. He lived for more than ten years with cancer, but my family knew that he didn't have much time left. The cancer became too much to bear, and there was no treatment that could extend his life.

As I lay in bed weeping and exhausted, my phone rang. I answered, and all I could hear was crying on the other line. No words needed to be exchanged—I knew exactly what that meant. My grandpa was gone. I called Dale, who was at dinner with his sister visiting from out of town. My plan was to wait until Dale got home to drive to my grandpa's house. I thought it would be best for him to stay at home while the baby slept, and that way he could continue visiting with his sister while she was in town.

Dale's plan was far different. He got home and just hugged me while I sobbed. Then he asked what he needed to pack for the baby. I told him he should stay with his sister and the baby. But that was absolutely not an option for him. So, we packed up the baby and all of us, including my sister-in-law, went to my grandpa's house. We stayed until three in the morning. I would have been perfectly content with Dale staying home with the baby, but he said he had to be there for me. He was able to stand alongside me and mourn with me.

Paul tells Christians that we must have the mentality of being there for one another. We must rejoice with and for one another. We must mourn with those who mourn. This is a powerful principle to live by in your marriage. As a couple, you should celebrate each other's achievements, accomplishments, and gifts. No matter how big or small the reason, choose to celebrate together. If one of you is winning, then you are both winning. If one of you has a reason to rejoice and celebrate, then you both do. The same is true of mourning and loss. If one of you is mourning the loss of a loved one, a job, a dream, or a relationship, then you both are. It may not directly affect your daily life, but if it affects your spouse, then it should matter.

Choosing to celebrate and mourn together gives you an opportunity to be the love of Jesus to your spouse.

Let's reflect: Think about the last time one of you came home with something to celebrate or with bad news. How was the reaction when you, or your spouse, heard the other's news? Is there a sense of mutual excitement when one of you wins in your relationship? Or does it often feel like one partner's victory is their own? If one of you is mourning the loss of something or someone in life, are you there for each other? And, if not, in what ways can you now choose to celebrate and/or mourn together?

OVERCOMING FAILURE

*When the Lord saw that he had gone over to look,
God called to him from within the bush, "Moses!
Moses!" And Moses said, "Here I am."*

—Exodus 3:4

Moses is often remembered for leading the Israelites out of
Egypt. There are children's songs dedicated to the victory of his
obedience and God using him to bring redemption to an entire
nation. If we could play a highlight reel of Moses's life, it would
show God speaking to him through a burning bush, the parting
of the Red Sea, and even manna raining down from Heaven. We
often forget about the failures in his life. The reason he fled Egypt
was because he killed a man. God knew about this and still chose
to speak his plan for Moses's life through a burning bush. This
was significant for Moses. In spite of his failures, God was going to
use him, and the burning bush event would forever be a significant reminder of this truth.

It would make sense for God to no longer use Moses
because not only did he kill a man, but he also did it in Egypt!
It seemed like a bad plan to use him for this job. This is actually
what made Moses so nervous. This was the very event that
reminded Moses of how unqualified he was for this task. There
came a moment when Moses needed to move past his own failure. God made it clear that he was going to use him, but Moses
had to first stop letting his past failures dictate his future.

The New Testament makes it clear that the same is true for us because of the blood of Jesus. Jesus gave of himself for us. There is no failure or blunder too large that makes us unusable by God. What if we flipped that and thought the same way about our marriages?

There will be individual and shared failures that can certainly define your marriage. You might both think God can no longer use you as a couple because of things that have happened. Now, I don't know what offenses have taken place. They may be just as big as you think they are, but please understand there is nothing too ugly and tragic for Jesus. He's not finished using your marriage. He's not done knitting the two of you together. He still wants to use your relationship for each other and for others. It's time to stop letting your past failures as a couple dictate your future. God did not bring the two of you together by accident. He has plans for what you will accomplish as a couple. He wants to use your relationship for the benefit of others and for the glory of his Kingdom.

God has not written you off because of your failures, and that means neither should you.

Let's put it into practice: Spend time talking together about what has hindered you from believing you can be used by God. Are there areas in church you'd like to serve together but think you don't measure up? Is there a couple you'd like to share your faith with but are afraid the failures in your marriage might push them away? I encourage you to bring these things before the Lord in prayer, then move forward in spite of your failures.

COMFORT IN THE UNKNOWN

But seek first his kingdom and his righteousness, and all these things will be given to you as well. Therefore do not worry about tomorrow, for tomorrow will worry about itself. Each day has enough trouble of its own.

—Matthew 6:33–34

I've always found great joy and pride in working. Even as a child, I had dreams of running a business, becoming a teacher, or even being a forensic scientist. Whenever someone would ask me about my desire to stay home with my future children, I always responded with, "I would like to continue working." Then came the day when I welcomed my oldest son into the world.

As time passed, I grew anxious about returning to work. It felt as if my heart was being ripped out of my chest, but the idea of no longer working also seemed unimaginable. I had no idea what a resolution even looked like. I began to pray for God to bring comfort to the pain in my heart. There were so many factors and even more unknowns. I began to plead for God to guide me and lead me as the desires of my heart were changing. I didn't want to be led by pure emotion. I genuinely wanted what was best for my family and even for my future long after my son is out of diapers.

There are any number of problems we are faced with regularly. Sometimes our dilemmas have an emotional, physical, or even mental impact. We usually find the greatest sense of relief in knowing the outcome or possible solutions. This is misplaced comfort. It's not really all that encouraging when the solution is something we don't like. The truest form of solace in the midst of the unknown is not in knowing the solution but knowing it's in Jesus. With Jesus, your comfort won't be lost when the solution is hard.

That's why Matthew writes about seeking Jesus and his righteousness rather than solutions. When our hearts are set on doing everything we can to seek Jesus, we will be filled with comfort. When you and your spouse are sitting in the midst of the unknown, set your eyes on Jesus. As you navigate what comes next and you take it step-by-step, choose to seek Jesus. I think we spend far too much time brainstorming and problem-solving when difficult situations come our way. We want to find the way to fix it, to arrive at the solution as quickly as possible. It would serve us better if we'd put an equal amount of energy into asking how to honor God in the process. He will guide you and your husband, but he will also be the source of your comfort.

Let's reflect: When a problem arises, how often do you and your spouse turn to Jesus? Are you more prone to talking through the factors you can control and the varying number of possibilities? Do you find the list of potential solutions brings you more comfort than praying about it? Together, pray to Jesus to be your source of comfort, then from that comfort, see what potential solutions Jesus has given to help solve the issues that have arisen.

MAKING SPACE FOR GRACE

*See to it that no one falls short of the grace of God
and that no bitter root grows up to cause trouble
and defile many.*

—Hebrews 12:15

Dale was making the grocery list, just as he does every Saturday morning. I was irritated that he continued to ask me, "What do you need from the grocery store?" I had a list of things I needed to get done that morning, with two crying children tugging on my legs who were dying of starvation, and I was figuring out what to make for breakfast. I had no space available to think about what we would be eating next week and what ingredients he should pick up. The truth is, Dale does much of the cooking, so I just needed to add snacks for the kids to the list. In my frustration, I told him to just go to the store, then I would figure out things on my end later.

A few hours later, the kids were fed. I had drunk my coffee and had eaten. When Dale returned from the store, I noticed a few of my favorite foods in the cabinet. It was so unexpected and certainly undeserved. Dale exercised unmerited favor for me and thought of me while at the grocery store. When I saw my favorite pan dulce sitting in the cabinet, my heart was warmed and apologetic toward my husband.

Grace goes a long way in marriage. Dale and I don't always get it right, but we try to extend grace as often and as much as we can to each other. The thing that's so hard about grace is that, by definition, it's undeserved. It isn't just nice to extend grace, but it's actually what God urges us to do. The writer of Hebrews tells us to never fall short of grace. He even goes on to say that a lack of grace makes room for bitterness to rise up.

It's easy to make room for bitterness and anger because they're more natural reactions. Grace is something you must be intentional about in your relationship. Love, tenderness, respect, and kindness will grow in your marriage when you make space for grace. Think of ways to extend favor to each other when you don't deserve it. Implementing this practice with each other will help bring your love for each other to the forefront. It will help stave off bitterness from taking root in your hearts and leading to a number of other relational issues. I've also found grace to be contagious. Receiving grace has a way of turning contentious situations around, causing you to want to extend grace in return. You will never regret making space for grace in your relationship.

Let's pray: Lord, extending grace is not a natural response, but I want it to be. Bring it to the forefront of our minds as often as possible. Help us be committed to show grace to each other. Amen.

FORGIVING EACH OTHER

*Bear with each other and forgive one another if any
of you has a grievance against someone. Forgive as
the Lord forgave you.*

—Colossians 3:13

One of the greatest skills you can develop in your relationship is forgiveness. It's also arguably one of the hardest skills. Learning how to be a good forgiver will change the entire course of your marriage. You will never run out of opportunities to extend and receive forgiveness. It doesn't matter how long you have been together, because there will always be ways big and small that you will hurt each other. Choosing forgiveness is not a dismissal of the hurt or pain but a decision not to retaliate.

Forgiveness is a foundational theme in Scripture and one every Christian is called to extend in their lives. In Colossians, Paul reminds us to forgive others as we have been forgiven by the Lord. There is no limit to God's forgiveness for us, so there should be no limit to our forgiveness for others. You should adopt and apply this same ethic in your marriage. There is no offense too large for you to forgive. Whenever I talk about forgiveness, I want to be sure to never suggest you continue to be placed in a situation of harm and offense. The biblical understanding of forgiveness should never be leveraged as a reason to stay in an abusive or unsafe relationship. The path to forgiveness should still be sought, but that doesn't mean it needs to be done within the confines of marriage.

Within your relationship, offenses should be discussed and worked through, but forgiveness should always be the end goal. This will strengthen your marriage and put your love into action. The sign of Jesus's love for us came in the form of forgiveness, and we can exemplify his forgiveness in our own relationships. Jesus's forgiveness also brings a lot of freedom within your relationship. The offender and offended are set free from the offense. Holding on to resentment of any kind is not healthy for you or your spouse. It will only lead to division and isolation.

Choosing forgiveness allows for wounds to be healed and gives opportunity for growth and honesty. In many ways, working through pain and an offense successfully will bind you closer together. It's not an easy process, which is why many choose to hold on to the resentment and pain. Holding on will only bring harm to your relationship.

Being committed to forgiveness may take on different forms depending on your marriage and the offense. It won't always happen overnight, and you might need to bring in outside help. There is absolutely no shame in taking these steps. In fact, it shows great strength to be willing to admit that there is a need for this in your relationship and that you are going to do whatever it takes to resolve the offense. God desires for your marriage to be a life-giving union, but that's impossible without the giving and receiving of forgiveness.

Let's put it into practice: The next time you or your spouse hurts each other, choose to talk about it. In this conversation, be empathetic and willing to listen to each other. If you are the offender, be apologetic and own your faults. If you have been offended, be honest about the situation and resist the temptation to hurt in return.

REFRESHING EACH OTHER

A generous person will prosper; whoever refreshes others will be refreshed.

—Proverbs 11:25

One piece of marriage advice has stuck with me throughout my own marriage: The relationship is never fifty-fifty all of the time. To expect that it is will bring only frustration, maybe even pain. I've personally seen this wisdom ring true in my marriage, and I've also seen the angst when I expect things to be fifty-fifty. This isn't to say you should expect either partner to carry more of the load in marriage than the other. I imagine if our relationships existed in a vacuum, then fifty-fifty would be a completely reasonable expectation, but that's not the case.

Your marriage is affected by many factors outside of your-selves. Things like work, schedules, friends, family, and even society have a way of impacting the way you move toward a healthy marriage. There will be days, weeks, and even seasons when your marriage looks more like sixty-forty or seventy-thirty. One of you might be caring for more of the daily household responsibilities or putting in more effort to stay connected. This is not ideal, and no marriage can stay in this state for too long without becoming dysfunctional. But there are times when one partner will carry more of a certain aspect in the marriage.

I can think of a recent example when this was the case with Dale and me. My job was entering into its busy season, which meant more hours and responsibilities for me. As I continued to give more to my work, I wasn't capable of doing many of the normal things at home. Things like cleaning up after Dale cooked dinner and spending a few hours watching our favorite show together after the kids went to bed were nearly impossible for me. So, Dale started cooking dinner and cleaning up afterward. This was a season when things were not fifty-fifty for our relationship. Again, there is no way we could continue to function this way indefinitely. However, for a season, we could make it work. It's in these moments of our marriage that we've had to commit to being generous to each other.

Oftentimes, we read about generosity in Scripture, and we think of money. In this week's proverb, we are encouraged to be generous with others for the sake of bringing refreshment. When you can both choose to be generous in your marriage, you are electing to refresh each other. There are any number of ways that you can pick to be generous with each other. It can be with your time, with the way you view each other in difficult situations, or even with the way you treat each other. Being generous means you give good things to each other freely and abundantly. What a wonderful way to mirror the gospel in your marriage as you give freely to each other.

Let's put it into practice: Over the next few days, find ways to be generous with each other. That might look like showing genuine affection or sending a text sharing how much you appreciate your spouse.

MINDFULLY PATIENT

Be completely humble and gentle; be patient,
bearing with one another in love.

—Ephesians 4:2

Both of my children have the amazing ability to go from being perfectly content to starving in five minutes. As I'm frantically scrambling to think about what I can quickly make that they will actually eat, my two boys often appear to be withering away from starvation. I hope these situations become less volatile as they get older and their brain stems develop, enabling them to better regulate their bodies and control their emotions. Until then, their ability to be patient under the circumstances is practically nonexistent.

As much as I like to joke about their lack of patience, I'm reminded that I'm not that much better. I catch myself asking Dale to take care of something, then ten minutes later becoming frustrated when my request still isn't fulfilled. I imagine you and your spouse have similar stories to tell.

The reality is that being patient is hard, and we have to be mindful of the moments when we are being impatient. I'm still learning how to be patient, and I catch myself lacking patience far more often than I'd like. It's so important to learn how to be patient in marriage.

The idea of exercising perseverance in the face of delay is learned. I imagine this is why the Bible has to remind us over and over again that we are to be patient people. In Paul's letter to the Ephesians, he describes what it looks like to be a mature believer, and one of these markers is patience. In the same way our faith should showcase humility, gentleness, unity, and love, we should also be patient.

In your marriage, this might look like exercising patience in the moment or over a longer period of time. You might have to be patient with each other as you adjust to different seasons in life. When one of you is stressed out about a situation at work and you see it spilling over into your marriage, be patient. When one of you is dealing with the loss of a loved one and the pain impacts the way you relate to each other, be patient. When one of you is having a hard time adjusting to anything going on in your lives, be patient. Some of these situations might require taking active steps toward healing. Or you may have to remove yourself from the situation all together. However it will happen, as you figure it out as a couple, continue to be patient.

Exercising patience often means you have to be mindful of the fact that you aren't being patient. Your love for each other will grow as you mindfully exercise patience toward each other.

Let's reflect: Do you find it easy to be patient with each other? What are some situations that bring out the impatience in either of you more than others? How can you mindfully exercise patience with each other in these situations?

VALUE EACH OTHER

Show proper respect to everyone, love the family of believers, fear God, honor the emperor.

—1 Peter 2:17

When Dale and I graduated from the seminary, we knew God had placed us together for a unique ministry opportunity. We didn't know what it would look like, but we talked about our desire to partner in ministry over and over again.

Out of these conversations, our blog and later podcast were born. Interesting enough, growing this ministry together has required us to learn each other's strengths and weaknesses rather quickly. Our ministry has seen the most growth when we've leaned in to the value each of us brings to the process. When it comes to the marketing and visionary side of our ministry, Dale is the expert. When it comes to managing and appealing to a wider range of backgrounds, I carry these strengths. There was a time when we didn't know the value each of us brought to the ministry, which made things challenging. We both became far happier understanding each other's value and knowing we are equally recognized.

A lack of honor, respect, and value brings friction to any relationship. In employee-employer relationships, respect is important from both parties. The same is true for family dynamics, in friendships, and in marriages. I can't think of any type of relationship that does not suffer when honor, respect, and value are not equally given and received. This is because all of humanity is created in the image of God.

All of us have an intrinsic value. With a high sense of value comes a need to be respected and honored. When relationships lack these things, there is fear, shame, isolation, and even anger. In Peter's first letter to the church, he's reminding Christians to show respect to everyone. He then goes on to expand on the idea of properly respecting others.

In your marriage, showing honor and respect toward each other should be assumed within your relationship. Viewing and treating each other as valuable—as individuals and in your marriage—is actually seeing each other as God created you. You should be able to speak to the unique value that each of you holds and to respect these aspects.

This can look like honoring each other's opinions and trusting the decisions you both make on behalf of the other. Value, honor, and respect must flow both ways. When this dynamic is established, your marriage will flourish because you are treating each other as God intended.

Let's pray: Heavenly Father, I pray we will continue to see each other as you see us, with value and dignity. I want us to always show each other respect and honor. Remind us to identify and cherish the unique value each of us brings into our relationship. Amen.

SUPPORT EACH OTHER'S GOALS

May he give you the desire of your heart and make all your plans succeed. May we shout for joy over your victory and lift up our banners in the name of our God. May the Lord grant all your requests.

—Psalm 20:4–5

When I was asked to write this book, although my first thought was "Yes," my second was "Is it possible?" Between working full-time from home, being the primary caretaker of our two children under two, and maintaining our ministry, it seemed like a tall task to take on another project. I talked with my husband about it, and after confirming this was something I wanted to do, he said, "We can do this." He was agreeing not only to support me in words but also to help make it possible for me to carve out time to write.

In our relationship, there are many things in our lives that we dream about and work toward together. But we also have dreams and goals that are separate from each other. I genuinely could not have completed this project if it weren't for Dale cheering me on and actively supporting me along the way.

In your marriage, it's healthy to have dreams of your own. And you should root for each other as if the dreams were your own. In Psalm 20, David writes about God granting the desires of your heart. The psalm is not about God operating as a wish granter but instead about God delighting in bringing about success in your life as you continue to seek him. As you set your eyes and heart on Jesus, the dreams and plans for your own life will fall in line with what he has in store for you. In the same way God wants to see your dreams come true in this context, we should long for the goals of our spouse to be accomplished.

Sometimes your dreams as individuals will feel like they cost you more than you'd like to pay. When your dreams or goals are in line with God, it's important that your marriage supports them. Remember what I said back in week 34 (page 68). As the two of you become one, it means that when one is winning, both of you are, and when one is succeeding, both of you are. You can both actively work toward helping each other accomplish your personal dreams and goals.

There should be a balance in your marriage, with both of you being able to dream and know you will support each other. Maintaining a team mentality is so important as you define what it means to be successful in your marriage. Supporting each other to achieve your dreams is about more than words—it often requires sacrifice for the sake of the health of your relationship as a whole.

Let's pray: Father, please give me the desire of your heart and make all your plans succeed. May we shout for joy over your victory and lift up our banners in the name of you. May you grant all my requests. Amen.

OVERCOMING TEMPTATIONS TOGETHER

No temptation has overtaken you except what is
common to mankind. And God is faithful; he will
not let you be tempted beyond what you can bear.
But when you are tempted, he will also provide a
way out so that you can endure it.

—1 Corinthians 10:13

I once heard a marriage described as a living organism that needs to be on guard against toxins that can cause infection. This is such a fitting analogy for the way temptation can creep into the life of a spouse and possibly cause the decline of a relationship.

The struggle with temptation on its own shouldn't be something to be ashamed of or feel guilty about. Everyone has something in their life that, if given a foothold, can bring about pain or turmoil. In Paul's first letter to the believers in Corinth, he addresses the reality of temptation in the life of every person. But he doesn't just tell us to be aware of these things. He actually gives hope to overcome temptation through the work of the Holy Spirit. The promise from God is not that temptation won't exist but that there will always be a way out. Each person has to make the decision to walk through the exit door instead of continuing down the enticing path of temptation. That's certainly much easier said than done.

When it comes to your marriage, you will both struggle with different types of temptations. What is a struggle for you may not be for your spouse and vice versa. Though you both have different challenges in this regard, you should be willing to overcome any of them as a couple. This might look like having a conversation about what you are struggling with and being honest about how hard it is for you to choose the exit door.

As a couple, you should feel safe sharing what is going on with you as an individual without fear of being judged by your spouse. It's also helpful to discuss clear boundaries regarding the temptations you're both struggling with. This could mean setting agreed-upon boundaries for how each of you interact with members of the opposite sex and a limit to how much alcohol you feel comfortable with each other consuming.

Practical systems to guard against temptation are wise, but we also can't neglect the power of turning to prayer. Create the boundaries both of you need, but also be dedicated to praying through any and all temptations you are struggling with. God will uphold his promise to provide an exit route out of temptation.

Let's reflect: Are you aware of the temptations both of you struggle with? Is your marriage a safe place to share when you are feeling compelled to act on your temptation? Are you open to your spouse sharing when they are concerned about a life choice that could lead to hardship in your marriage? If you answered no to any of these questions, choose a time when you and your spouse can have an open and honest conversation about your struggles, making your marriage a safe space, and how to share any concerns about life choices either of you are thinking of making.

HAVING A VOICE

The way of fools seems right to them, but the wise listen to advice.

—Proverbs 12:15

When I was engaged, I had a conversation with a newly married woman, which made me fearful about what I was about to commit my life to. She shared about wanting to save up for a house, and her husband had proposed they move in with his mother. She was on the verge of tears as she described how terrible this idea felt to her and the complexities of her relationship with her mother-in-law. Things were messy, and the idea of moving in with her mother-in-law was the last thing she wanted to do. It truly brought her great anxiety.

In a later conversation, I asked her what decision she and her husband had made about their living situation. She waited several moments before sharing that they would be moving in with her mother-in-law despite her pleading for another option. My heart sank as I wondered if this was what all marriages are like.

Making decisions within a marriage can be a huge challenge, especially when spouses are not seeing eye to eye. At the end of the day, a decision has to be made and life needs to go on, but it shouldn't be without the consideration of both spouses. To have one spouse dominate every decision with no regard for the impact the decision will have on the marriage as a whole is unwise. In Proverbs 12, we are reminded that a fool will always see their way as the right way, and they will open neither their ears nor their hearts to any other way or opinion.

To shut out the voice of one member in the marriage is harmful to the relationship and to the individual. As a couple, you should be committed to allowing both voices to be heard, to be considered, and to have equal weight. It is destructive to make one person in the marriage feel as if they have no say in the outcome of their own life. In extreme cases, this level of control can be considered abusive behavior, as one spouse is essentially ruling and dominating the other spouse.

Healthy marriages allow for, and even require, both voices to be equal in value, weight, and importance. A marriage is made up of two people with two perspectives and desires that must be heard. If one voice is not heard or taken into consideration, it can lead to bitterness and resentment within the relationship. Allowing both voices to be heard might be more challenging and take added time, effort, and energy to work through decisions. But this approach will maintain the health and happiness of your marriage. Allowing both voices to speak about a situation can lead to a far better outcome for everyone involved rather than deeming one person's opinion as the only right decision. Giving each other a voice in your relationship adds value and dignity to your marriage.

Let's reflect: How does your relationship function when you have different opinions about major decisions? Do both of you have an equal voice, or does one carry more weight than the other? If both voices are not equal, how can you and your spouse begin the work to equalize?

A COMMITMENT TO TRUTH

Do not lie to each other, since you have taken off your old self with its practices and have put on the new self, which is being renewed in knowledge in the image of its Creator.

—Colossians 3:9–10

Just about everyone would agree it's important not to lie. It is a life value most people are taught from a very young age. Lies have a way of causing relationships to shatter from within. When a lie is uncovered, the entire relationship is called into question. I imagine you are nodding your head and thinking to yourself that this isn't a revolutionary idea. It's not. But as simple as this truth is, and as much as we all know it, many of us tend to push honesty aside when we find ourselves in situations in which a little white lie could quickly get us out.

One of the markers of a person receiving faith in Jesus is transformation. There is an instantaneous transformation of the state of your soul at the moment of salvation, and there is an ongoing transformation of your heart and mind as you grow in your faith. One of the areas in which we should transform as believers is in our willingness to lie to others.

In Colossians, we are told the practice of lying is something we did in our old nature, but we were made new in Jesus. Lying should no longer be part of who we are. This old nature should not have a home in our hearts, actions, or relationships. As we desire for our marriage to reflect our Creator, we should commit to keeping it free of lies. Even the smallest of lies can sow seeds of doubt and deception, which can destroy your relationship from the inside out.

Oftentimes, we'd rather lie than bring to light a flaw, an error, or a sin to the person we love. As much as you think you are pre-serving your marriage by lying—no matter how minor—you are only prolonging the inevitable damage that will ensue. You might even be causing more damage in the long run.

In a relationship marked by lies and deception, God can bring restoration and healing. Certain lies may have caused so much damage and pain that you are unsure of how your marriage can continue. In these situations, it's important not to take general principles as the rule that you must abide by, but rather seek pro-fessional and spiritual help in order to give you biblical wisdom for your very specific circumstance.

If your marriage affirms or makes accommodations for *small* lies, I encourage you and your spouse to make a shift, a transfor-mation. I urge you to remember Colossians. Think of lying as "the old nature" and implement the words of Paul, agreeing not to lie to each other. Adopting the commitment to never lie to each other strengthens your marriage to endure some of the most challenging situations it will face.

Let's reflect: Does your marriage make accommodations for small lies? If so, why do you think that is? How has the accom-modation helped or hurt your relationship? What would it look like to build a marriage free of all lies? Is this a conversation you would be willing to have with each other?

ALWAYS GROWING

The righteous will flourish like a palm tree,
they will grow like a cedar of Lebanon; planted
in the house of the Lord, they will flourish in the
courts of our God. They will still bear fruit in old
age, they will stay fresh and green, proclaiming,
"The Lord is upright; he is my Rock, and there
is no wickedness in him."

—Psalm 92:12–15

When it comes to babies, growth is always celebrated. But when that baby grows into adulthood, our mentality toward growth shifts to hesitancy and sometimes fear. There is a point when we just want to be comfortable in life, and usually growth means stepping into a state of uncomfortableness. I wish growth could happen apart from uncertainty, pain, and uncomfortableness, but that's not how it works. Growing pains are very real, and they aren't only limited to our bodies. As we think about where to grow in our marriages, it begins with growth in the individual. That can be scary.

I've often thought about my own marriage and the ways Dale's and my perspectives, thoughts, and passions have changed in the last few years. If I think too long about this, I can allow myself to become fearful of our individual journeys of growth. I've heard of marriages growing apart as the individuals changed from who they were when they first met.

It's so important that we never stop growing, but it's equally important that, for a marriage to last and work, we grow in the same direction. There has to be something guiding and directing a couple's growth for them to remain connected and knitted together. However, the reality of growing apart is real, and unfortunately it happens to many couples. But growing apart doesn't have to happen, and truly it shouldn't. The answer is not to reject all growth but rather to stay committed to the people you were when you first met. It would be a tragedy to look back on your marriage and realize neither of you have grown over the course of ten, twenty, or thirty years.

Growth is a good thing and should be encouraged in your marriage, but you have to stay committed to growing in the same direction. Psalm 92 describes the people of God flourishing, growing, and becoming sturdy like trees. The picture being painted in this verse is that the people of God can grow in the right direction only when they are firmly planted in him.

Do not fear growth in your marriage. In fact, be committed to growth together, in the right direction. When both of you continue to be firmly planted in God, then you have nothing to fear as you grow as individuals and as a couple. You will find your roots grow deeper into your faith as you surround yourself with believers. Study the Word of God and allow yourself to be led by the Holy Spirit. This is where growth happens. With this as your foundation, you can look forward to flourishing. Even the fruit your marriage will bear will be for the Kingdom of God.

Let's put it into action: When was the last time you stepped outside of your comfort zone? Is there a way you can commit to growing deeper in your faith as individuals and as a couple?

A LOVE FOR GOD

*"Love the Lord your God with all your heart and
with all your soul and with all your mind and with
all your strength."*

—Mark 12:30

One of the most fundamental principles to the Christian faith is a love for God. From the Old to the New Testaments, we are called to love God and to love others. Everything about Christianity boils down to these two things, so to not have them is to not have the Christian faith. Your love for God must be fundamental to your very life and everything that flows out of it. This includes your marriage.

Seeing your marriage grow and flourish can't happen apart from a commitment to loving God. As you both set your heart, mind, and soul on loving the Lord more deeply, you will find you grow in your ability to love each other better.

Mark describes the command to love God as all-encompassing. You can't merely love God with your heart and not your mind. God doesn't want to be the focus of a certain section of your life—he wants all of you so that he can redeem all of you. It is your love for Christ that binds you together.

When your eyes are focused on Jesus, everything else will change. The way you think will change. Your understanding of your role on this earth will be for the glory of God. The greatest challenges you face can be met with the strength of Jesus, which will fuel your ability to push forward. Out of your love for Jesus, everything else will flow. In your journey of transformation to be more like Jesus, you will find your marriage becoming more like

Jesus as well. The goal is not to love Jesus with the sole intent of your marriage growing. Certainly, as you center your life on Jesus, growth in your marriage will be a natural byproduct.

As both partners desire to love Jesus more and more, you will increase your love for each other. Out of Jesus's forgiveness for you and the great offenses committed in your life, you can better extend forgiveness in your marriage. When you've seen the overwhelming love Jesus has for you and what it means to be loved for who you are, then you can give the same kind of love in your relationship. When you place growing your love for Jesus at the center of your life, the impacts for your marriage will be greater than you ever could have imagined.

Let's pray: God, I know my journey to loving you more is ongoing. I have not arrived at what it means to truly love you with every part of me. There have been times when my love for you was all I could see, and there have been times when it was buried in the back of my mind under all of the other things happening around me. I ask that my love for you and my spouse's love for you would be the focus of our marriage. Amen.

FREE OF COMPARISON

Each one should test their own actions. Then they can take pride in themselves alone, without comparing themselves to someone else, for each one should carry their own load.

—Galatians 6:4–5

There are many great benefits to building virtual communities. There are also some real downsides. One of my current favorite virtual groups is full of moms with children the same age as my boys. It's so fun to see fellow mothers posting pictures of their little one reaching exciting and challenging milestones. It's also a place to be honest about the struggles of parenting or to ask questions about whether or not all the other moms are experiencing the same thing. I'm so grateful for this community and the many ways it has helped ground me in reality.

One major downside to the group is the temptation toward comparison. I found myself being less excited about the achievements and growth my boys were having when I saw how advanced other children were. I would be so proud of the language development of my two-year-old, until I read about a one-year-old speaking in whole sentences. What was supposed to be a joyous moment turned into questions of doubt and concern.

Comparison is a real struggle many of us have to deal with. We look at the other people around us who are similar in age, life stage, or background and wonder why or how they are doing better in life than we are. Maybe it's a friend from high school who just posted on social media about purchasing her first home and it's a beachfront property. You want to be excited for her, but it's so hard when your success doesn't match hers. Whether it's celebrating the milestones significant to you, achieving the goal you set out to do, or rising up through challenging times, it will always seem like there is someone you know personally or virtually who is doing better. This is when the frustration of comparison sneaks in.

Comparison will bring only destruction and rob you of joy. When it comes to your marriage, it's extremely helpful to guard your heart against comparing your relationship with others. The success, happiness, and enjoyment of your marriage is not dependent on another couple. Whether or not another couple seems to be more in love, handling life better, or managing marital challenges better doesn't mean your relationship is failing.

In the book of Galatians, we are called to stay focused on our own work and to even be proud of what we've done without comparing ourselves with our neighbor. For us today, this means keeping our eyes focused on our marriage and not comparing it with those of our friends on Instagram or the other woman at church. You should both be proud of the hard work you've put into your marriage and the growth you've experienced. Don't allow comparison to rob you of the joy God wants you to have.

Let's reflect: When was the last time you compared your relationship with another couple? Maybe you saw the way a husband treated his wife and wished your interactions were the same. You may be longing to be as put together as another wife or fiancé you saw on Instagram. How can you commit to removing comparison with others from your marriage?

GENEROSITY-BASED MARRIAGE

Remember this: Whoever sows sparingly will also reap sparingly, and whoever sows generously will also reap generously.

—2 Corinthians 9:6

There are many inwardly focused areas that married and engaged couples should focus on to keep growing together. Areas like intimacy, thoughtfulness, and quality time are quickly thought of when it comes to finding places to strengthen your marriage. It's not as common for us to view outwardly focusing areas as ways to grow closer together. Yet there is something about coming together to care for the needs of others that will actually bond you and your spouse together.

The Bible talks about the act of generosity as something that will benefit those who are generous. One of those verses is found in 2 Corinthians. Paul is essentially telling believers that what you are willing to give will also be what you receive. If you cling tightly to all of the blessings and resources you've been given, without thinking of ways to share them with others, then you will likely see these things remain scarce in your life.

It is important to note that Paul isn't suggesting that God is withholding from you because you haven't given enough. This verse should be viewed as a piece of biblical advice and not as a biblical promise. If you are not in a place of abundance, it doesn't necessarily mean it's because you've been stingy. If you are in a place of prosperity, it doesn't necessarily mean you've been an extremely generous person. This verse is not describing a one-to-one correlation between generosity and prosperity and stinginess and lacking.

The verse expresses a common piece of wisdom that if you are generous, then you will likely see generosity be given in return. As a couple, you should desire to be as generous as you can with the things God has given you. This means you should view all things you've been given as a reminder to give back to others. When your heart desires to be generous, you may be surprised at the ways in which you are filled and blessed.

Generosity doesn't always require finances. You might be able to commit to being generous with your time, space, and even relationships. The ways in which you choose to express generosity to others can be big or small. It might look like making your home available to host a meal for your neighbors or opening your doors to be a place for your church's youth group to gather. Maybe it looks like being generous with your weekends by committing to serving in your church or offering to babysit a friend's kids so they can have a date night. This may not seem all that beneficial to your marriage, but coming together to give of yourself to others will strengthen your bond. There are likely far more ways for you to be generous if you are both on board, rather than just one member of the marriage.

Let's reflect: *Do you view your marriage as an opportunity to be generous to others? What would it look like for both of you to lean in to generosity in a way you currently are not?*

LEAVING A LEGACY TOGETHER

One generation commends your works to another;
they tell of your mighty acts.

—Psalm 145:4

I work for a nonprofit that's primarily funded by people who are in their sixties and seventies. I've often wondered why it is that people within this age category are more likely to financially support a nonprofit like the one I work for. There are certainly varying factors, but a main factor is that people within this age category are more apt to think about giving to something that will make an impact long after they are gone. They want to leave a legacy that is bigger than themselves. Every Christian, regardless of age, should be thinking of the next generations and being intentional about leaving a legacy of Christ.

When it comes to your marriage, leaving a legacy should be a focus of how you orchestrate your lives. As a couple, you should be mindful and intentional about leaving a legacy for the next generation. Your legacy may look different depending on your interests as a couple and the resources made available to you. Through your relationship, you can work toward the mission of Jesus to share your faith and make disciples. This mission is meant to impact the next generation.

God chooses people to make his name known, which means one generation telling another. In Psalm 145, the author writes about one generation telling the next about the works of God so that they would know him and believe. This should be a burden our souls and marriages carry, to tell the next generation about the works of God. This is not merely the mission of pastors and ministers but of every Christian.

The legacy you and your spouse leave might look like raising children in the ways of the Lord. But that is not the only way to leave a legacy. There are any number of ways to share, teach, and model your faith in Christ to the next generation. As you are around younger people and finding ways to serve them, you can both show them what a godly marriage looks like. You can share about your faith and the way God has continued to knit you together. Part of the purpose of your marriage is to leave a legacy for Jesus together. God brought the two of you together for your good but also for the good of others. Your marriage has a purpose that will impact more than just the two of you—it can make an impact for those who come after you, too.

Let's put it into action: Are you both intentional about impacting the next generation? If you have children, how can you show them the light of Christ in new ways? If you don't have children, how can you commit to interacting with the next generation? Decide on one activity you will do as a couple to reach, interact, or serve the next generation for Jesus.

FINDING THE GOODNESS IN MARRIAGE

*Two are better than one, because they have a good
return for their labor: If either of them falls down,
one can help the other up. But pity anyone who falls
and has no one to help them up.*

—Ecclesiastes 4:9–10

It's no secret that marriage is hard work. For some couples joining life with another person comes easily, but for many it is a transition and even a challenge. As much as you love each other, merging together two lives takes adjusting and a lot of sacrifice. Marriage can't be all about one spouse serving the other. It takes a mutual agreement to dedicate your heart, soul, and mind to the benefit and health of the one you love. When both couples operate from this philosophy, marriage can truly be enjoyed as God intended.

One of the many benefits that accompany the institution of marriage is found in Ecclesiastes 4. The ancient wisdom of two being better than one still holds up today. There is great practical benefit when two people work in the same direction. A lot more can be accomplished when there are double the set of hands. But marriage is about more than operating efficiently, though that's also not something to brush to the side. There is a benefit to having a built-in partner to care for you when you're down, cheer you on every step of the way, and lift you up when you fall. There are countless great relationships God has designed for us to engage in, but none are like marriage.

There are numerous resources out there, which provide wisdom on navigating the difficulties of marriage. However, what many of them lack is the reminder that there are also many benefits to marriage. The union you've made as a couple can be something you truly find joy and comfort in for years and years. It doesn't always have to be a relationship that is full of challenges. Each of you can grow in strength, love, grace, and understanding as a result of your marriage. God will use your marriage to sanctify you, but he will also use it to bring you joy. There should be an element of sheer excitement within your marriage because of the union formed between you. I imagine that as you look back to your wedding day, you remember being excited to marry your spouse. That same type of excitement to do life with each other should be there.

As you continue to grow in your marriage and to build a godly union, don't forget to take time to see the many benefits and joy your marriage brings.

Let's pray: Lord, thank you for the ways you have already grown my marriage. Help us see your goodness in the day-to-day things. Encourage us when we feel defeated by the challenges, and remind us of the many benefits and joy that we bring to each other. Amen.

RELENTLESS LOVE

My command is this: Love each other as I have loved you.

—John 15:12

There is one story in the Bible that has always made me a bit uncomfortable because of what its implications are in my own life. It is the story of Hosea. His display of love reminds me how often my love for Dale falls short of what God has called me to.

If you are unfamiliar with the story of Hosea, God calls this man to prophesize to the people in Northern Israel. He is to bring to light the ways they have turned away from God and share that there is still hope for them to turn back to God.

What is so difficult about this story is that Hosea's marriage is a prophetic symbol of God's love for his people. Hosea is married to a woman named Gomer who is unfaithful to him multiple times. They have three children together in the midst of Gomer being unfaithful, and the marriage begins to fall apart. Hosea goes out to find his wife, pay off her debts to her lovers, and recommit his love to her. He pursues his wife again, in spite of the pain and stress she has caused their marriage.

The destruction and restoration of Hosea's marriage is used as an image of what God has done for his people. In spite of his people turning away from him, God continues to pursue his people to bring them back to himself. God pursues his people out of his own compassion, faithfulness, and love for them. This is exactly what he has done for you and me. It doesn't matter how great your offenses toward God have been, how dark your past may be, or even how much hurt you have caused; the love of Jesus covers all of this. His love for you is greater than the worst thing you have ever done. This is how God loves you.

When we put into perspective the way in which we are loved by God, a verse like John 15:12 has a heavy meaning. In this verse, we are commanded to love others as God has loved us. In our marriages, we are expected to love each other relentlessly.

Now, I want to be clear in saying that if your spouse is unfaithful in your marriage, the story of Hosea and Gomer is not necessarily the case study for how you are supposed to bring restoration. However, the life of Hosea is meant to show us what God's love looks like. Even in marriage, we are to love each other as Jesus has loved us. This can be a hard call sometimes. It can mean choosing to work through the hurts and pains caused by each other for the sake of love and restoration. It can mean extending kindness and grace when your spouse doesn't deserve it. Jesus's love for you is the best model for how you are to give and receive love in your marriage.

Let's reflect: How would you describe the giving and receiving of love in your marriage? What would change if both of you committed to loving each other relentlessly in every aspect of your relationship, loving each other in the way God loves you?

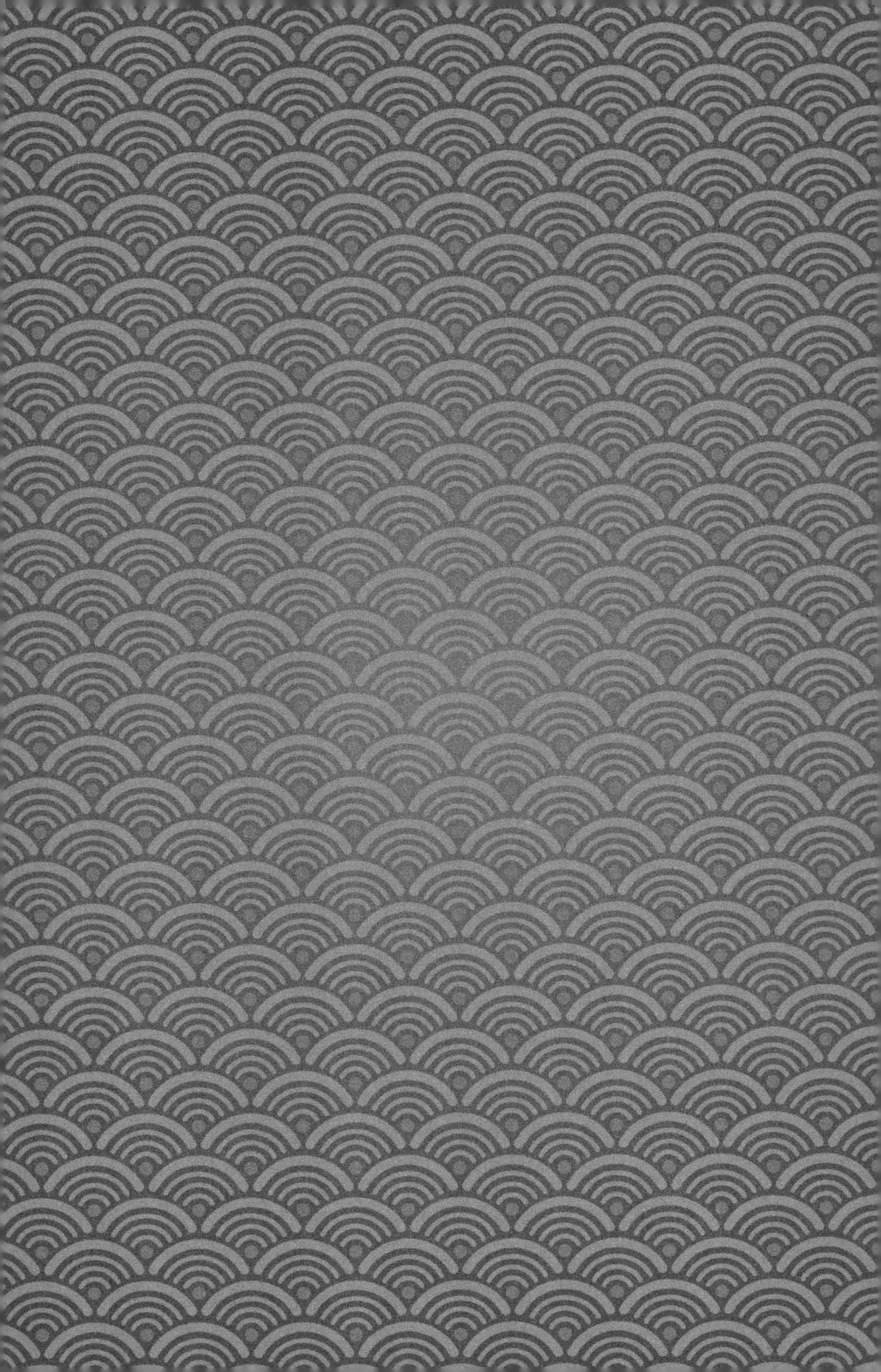

ACKNOWLEDGMENTS

Many thanks to my husband, Dale, for your ongoing commitment to love me more and more. You always have a way of believing in me even when I don't. I pray our sons see a glimmer of Jesus's love as they watch us love each other.

ABOUT THE AUTHOR

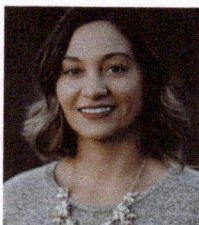

Tamara Chamberlain is a writer and podcaster who is passionate about helping people wrestle with how to live the high calling Jesus has given them in everyday life. Her other books are *Prayers for Your Future Husband* and *Practicing Christian Compassion*. She holds a master of divinity from Talbot School of Theology and lives in California with her husband, Dale, and their two sons. You can connect with Tamara at HerAndHymn.com.

CPSIA information can be obtained
at www.ICGtesting.com
Printed in the USA
JSHW040452010322
23360JS00003B/3

9 781638 072072